The Problems and Prospects of LSD

(Third Printing)

The Problems and Prospects of LSD

Edited by

J. THOMAS UNGERLEIDER, M.D.

Assistant Professor of Psychiatry
UCLA Center for the Health Sciences
Los Angeles, California

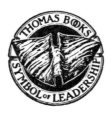

CHARLES C THOMAS • PUBLISHER
Springfield • Illinois • U.S.A.

Published and Distributed Throughout the World by
CHARLES C THOMAS • PUBLISHER
BANNERSTONE HOUSE
301-327 East Lawrence Avenue, Springfield, Illinois, U.S.A.
NATCHEZ PLANTATION HOUSE
735 North Atlantic Boulevard, Fort Lauderdale, Florida, U.S.A.

© *1968 by* CHARLES C THOMAS • PUBLISHER
ISBN 0-398-01952-5
Library of Congress Catalog Card Number: 68-18308

First Printing, 1968
Second Printing, 1970
Third Printing, 1972

With THOMAS BOOKS *careful attention is given to all details of manufacturing and design. It is the Publisher's desire to present books that are satisfactory as to their physical qualities and artistic possibilities and appropriate for their particular use.* THOMAS BOOKS *will be true to those laws of quality that assure a good name and good will.*

Printed in the United States of America
N-1

CONTRIBUTORS

SIDNEY COHEN, M.D. is Chief of Psychosomatic Medicine, Veteran's Administration Hospital, Los Angeles, and Associate Clinical Professor of Medicine at UCLA. His area of research interest is psychopharmacology with over ninety papers published, of which some twenty-five articles and two books deal with LSD.

KEITH DITMAN, M.D. is Research Psychiatrist and Lecturer, Department of Psychiatry, UCLA School of Medicine. He is consultant on drugs to the American Medical Association and has authored three books and approximately seventy publications, mostly in the area of psychopharmacology. He has been working with LSD for the past ten years and currently is principal investigator on one of the largest clinical studies with LSD in the country, evaluating LSD as a treatment for alcoholism.

DUKE FISHER, M.D. is Psychiatric Resident at the Neuropsychiatric Institute, UCLA Medical Center. He has lectured widely, authored several articles, and contributed chapters to several books, all on LSD. He has done extensive work in the area of side effects and treatment of complications from LSD.

JOEL FORT, M.D. is Lecturer, Department of Sociology, University of California, Davis; and developer and former Director, Center for Special Problems, San Francisco Health Department; former Consultant on Drug Abuse,

World Health Organization and the United Nations; and co-author of *Utopiates,* Atherton Press, 1964.

J. THOMAS UNGERLEIDER, M.D. is Assistant Professor of Psychiatry, UCLA Center for the Health Sciences. He has authored over twenty-five articles and contributed chapters on LSD to half a dozen books. His special area of interest is the side effects from LSD, as seen both in hospitals and in the community.

To John and Peggy, and to adolescents now and in the future—may theirs not be a *drugged* solution to life's problems.

PREFACE TO THE THIRD PRINTING

In the interim since the first printing of this book, the drug abuse situation has continued to deteriorate in the United States. With the "death" of the Flower children in 1967 in the Haight-Ashbury district, the situation changed from one of use of the strong psychedelics, particularly LSD, as part of a life style by an older age group, to the chronic multiple, indiscriminate use of many types of drugs by younger and younger persons. Reports of widespread drug use in junior high schools, and even reports of use in elementary schools, are being presented with increasing frequency. In some states like California, schools are beginning educational programs about drugs as early as kindergarten. President Nixon has called drug abuse our number one problem and has created a Special Action Office to coordinate all federal efforts and to increase funds available and number and kinds of programs offered.

Not only have younger people continued to experiment with the amphetamines and barbiturates and a wide variety of fad drugs, but heroin has now "hit" the affluent areas, which defies all rational thought and comprehension. Methadone maintenance programs have received wide publicity. The drug abuse scene is "where the action is." Political leaders say it's suicide politically to be against any drug abuse program. Evaluation of the effectiveness of programs in control/enforcement, prevention/education and treatment/rehabilitation, however, still remains most difficult.

As for LSD itself, it has fallen somewhat out of vogue because of the widespread street dissemination of knowledge of the unpredictability of this powerful substance, because of the highly publicized but much disputed "chromosome damage" and because the pure "Owsley's Acid or Stanley's Stuff" that was available in 1965 is no longer available. Much sold on the street is adulterated with contaminants or is not LSD at all. Because LSD is not widely sought (100,000 tablets of pure potent LSD were confiscated in a western city recently, selling for 15 cents a tablet because they were sold as LSD), a number of other drugs which contain LSD are sold, purportedly as other compounds. Mescaline is a particular favorite now, particularly if termed "organic" and, thus (the mythology goes) a natural and safe experience. But of two hundred cases of alleged mescaline recently analyzed in a Northern California Free Clinic, not one was found to contain it. *All* of our samples of alleged mescaline which have been analyzed contain either LSD or phencyclidine, the veterinary anesthetic. An LSD taboo has thus been added to the heroin and needle taboos.

Federal legislation has been changing, more to focus punitive and deterrent controls on the seller or "pusher" rather than on the user. In May of 1971, it became a misdemeanor *federally* for simple first-time possession of small amounts of all dangerous drugs, including LSD. Approximately twenty-five states have adopted this Uniform Drug Act, to date, with more expected to do so soon.

Unfortunately, research into LSD has all but been discontinued and the therapeutic effects, particularly using LSD in psychotherapy and in dying patients, remain unknown. Hundreds of films have been made about the drug abuse problem, many referring to LSD, and evaluation of these is being done by several national agencies and one young people's student group (Project DARE, at UCLA in Los Angeles). Unfortunately, some, in their zeal to dissuade youngsters from attempting experimentation and use of drugs, have taken the fact that marijuana is regarded by some as a mild psychedelic and have attributed all LSD's potential adverse reactions to the cannabis derivatives. This has had a backlash effect which limits and further reduces credibility: So often heavy users of multiple drugs say: "They lied to us about marijuana and we figured they were lying about acid (LSD), coke (cocaine), speed (methamphetamine) and smack (heroin) too." Wide controversy today seems focused on the continued criminalization of users, particularly of the cannabis derivatives. Indeed, a National Commission (of which the editor is a member) was created several months ago by Congress and appointed by the President to study the drug abuse problem, focusing on cannabis in the first year and the other drugs of abuse in the second year.

LSD has figured predominantly in a number of trials, particularly for mass murder, on the West Coast. In a rather sensational fashion, psychiatrists have testified both for and against the ability of the drug to rob the person of knowledge and intent to formulate the act of murder. In other words, LSD psychosis is being used as a defense against murder. An LSD-treated potato chip party created havoc and received great publicity in Los Angeles recently and resulted in a long jail term for the "prankster." A new nickname has been claimed for LSD, and that is "Let's Simmer Down" (i.e. a plea for less hysteria).

Another focus in the drug scene has been on *meaningful alternative* experiences involving youth who have been experimenting with these drugs, particularly in terms of creating peer groups where it is "in" not to use drugs, and in terms of self-esteem building activities via work, interpersonal relationships and artistic pursuits. Hot lines and Free Clinics have proliferated as physicians have been reluctant to come forward to treat the drug abuser in traditional facilities.

On the bleak side, currently in California, two physicians

(AMA members) are being investigated by the Board of Medical Examiners via a hearing through the Attorney-general's office for withdrawing heroin abusers in a private hospital with *non*-narcotics like Mellaril. An ancient California law states that no narcotic addict may be treated except in an approved (county, university or veteran's, etc.) hospital. In the past, this rule was interpreted to mean no heroin addict may be treated with methadone; but now, under literal interpretation, and because marijuana (and cocaine and peyote) is a narcotic under California statute, and because the word *addiction* is being defined as drug dependence, both *psychologic* and *physiologic,* no marijuana-dependent person, for example, may legally be treated in any way (with psychotherapy, drug therapy or as an outpatient) by any therapist or physician. This tragedy, of course, is totally counter to the thrust of Mr. Nixon's entire efforts to provide treatment of those who seek and need help, as well as the efforts of professionals and even many law enforcement groups.

But so symbolic and so intense are the emotions about drugs, that failure to insure adequate treatment facilities without reporting users to the police has driven many young people from the established facilities and into the free "hippie" clinics. Thus, the situation looks both hopeful and bleak at the same time. The public is aroused and beyond hysteria, and no longer is the one-shot "famous lecturer" in the school the way communities are planning to effectively handle the drug problem. Rather, they're realizing that a concerted effort by all groups, including law enforcement, educators, parents, physicians and other helpers, the ministry and business executives, is needed to combat this symptomatic piece of behavior known as drug abuse. Attention is also beginning to be paid to differentiation of drug use and abuse, as both terms are not synonomous (100 million people use alcohol but we have "only" 10 million alcoholics in this country) .

Must we not make the same differentiation between use and abuse of the other drugs like marijuana, amphetamines, barbiturates, etc., too?

Must we not also consider the use of drugs for pleasure, not only under the guise of medical prescription?

As a footnote, I have just returned from a tour of the Far and Middle East with the Marijuana Commission and in almost every country we heard that wherever the hippies go (not only or even primarily American hippies), the psychedelic drugs like LSD are introduced. But in these countries, the primary problem of major consequence is the opium-heroin problem; thus the LSD phenomenon seems to be of affluent countries.

J. T. L.

PREFACE TO THE FIRST PRINTING

One of the most powerful drugs today is d-lysergic acid diethylamide tartrate, commonly called LSD or, by users, "acid" or "L." It is extremely difficult to provide a comprehensive picture of the LSD situation in one volume, for several reasons. The first has to do with the "LSD hysteria" in which we find ourselves today. There has been so much written and aired about LSD, a great deal of which has been seductive publicity, that we have a great deal of misinformation on both sides. For example, I have received literature that all LSD used in the United States is a Communist plot. I receive letters that God will strike me dead for *not* recommending LSD to everyone. LSD was a political issue in the last California governor's race. We have heard it implicated in everything from police brutality to the Vietnam situation. Proponents of the drug, who insist that it offers instant happiness, instant creativity in art or music, and instant fame for architects now vie with the total disclaimers who insist that LSD is more dangerous than heroin, that it should be outlawed completely, including research, and that all proponents like Dr. Timothy Leary should be prevented from speaking or even advertising in newspapers.

Another factor which increases the difficulty in understanding the LSD problem is that the picture is constantly changing. Originally, LSD difficulties were common among chronic drug abusers, but now we are increasingly seeing youngsters who experimented once with the drug, got over the acute effects and then a number of months later began to have reoccurrences of the original symptoms without ever taking the drug again. And LSD-induced amnesia (a rare, if ever, occurring phenomenon) is now being claimed as a defense against robbery and murder.

The one legitimate manufacturer of the drug, Sandoz Laboratories, discontinued production of LSD approximately two years ago and turned over all existing supplies of the drug to the National Institute of Mental Health. Thus almost all obtainable LSD has become black market manufactured and many researchers subsequently left the field of LSD research with the vital questions about this most powerful drug still unanswered.

Unfortunately, the use of the drug among the population increases steadily. Where LSD was originally used mainly by professionals, intellectuals and artistic people, its use now has spread to the colleges, high schools, junior high schools and to all socioeconomic groups.

So much for the situation surrounding LSD today. In this volume we will begin with the consideration of LSD as one drug among a number of other drugs which are used and abused, particularly in the United States. We will also learn about the history of LSD and other hallucinogens in general.

Then we will review the research aspects of LSD. These have to do with administration of the pure drug to subjects who have been screened by psychiatric interview and psychological testing, with measurement of resultant subjective and/or objective effects. Next we will describe the therapy employing LSD with various kinds of patients. This is a highly challenging field of great potential and, at the present time, also one of no little controversy.

Following this we will consider the acute and chronic side effects from LSD. This is an area where a great deal of misinformation exists and where an entire "LSD mythology" has arisen, partly in order to explain away the helpless situation in which the LSD user who begins to have "a freak trip" finds himself. Then finally we will consider the prospects of LSD—its future possibilities. The contributors have different points of view, and the reader will note marked controversy between them. But it is only by examining the various positions that a more rational view of the LSD problem may emerge.

J. THOMAS UNGERLEIDER, M.D.

INTRODUCTION

This monograph is an outgrowth of a breakfast panel entitled "The Problems and Potential of LSD," which was held in Las Vegas at the American Medical Association's Clinical Convention. The same five participants on that panel, each with his special interest and experience in a different area of LSD work, are the contributors to this volume.

All of the contributors have previously written about LSD, and all have been consultants to or have testified before gubernatorial, state or national legislative bodies on the problems of LSD. All the panelists are also from California, the state that leads the nation in so many things, like the LSD problem.

CONTENTS

The Problems and Prospects of LSD

Chapter I

LSD AND THE MIND-ALTERING DRUG (M.A.D.) WORLD

JOEL FORT

"From out of the city the dying groan, and the soul of the wounded cries for help."

BOOK OF JOB

"He who tries to determine everything by law will foment crime rather than lessen it."

SPINOZA

INTRODUCTION

In *Utopiates*, which I co-authored in 1964, I stated, "It seems highly probable that greater and excessive controls of legitimate medical and scientific use, exaggerated statements, increasing illicit use, and discouragement of scientific research will occur in the coming years." Unhappily, that prediction was accurate, and in fact, the present sensationalism, hysteria and fanaticism exceed the expectations of all but the most cynical and pessimistic. It has been truly said that those who do not learn from the past are doomed to repeat it, and our society has learned nothing from the previous failures of the American system of drug control, first with alcohol, then with narcotics, and more recently with marijuana. Understanding and solving any problem depends upon a proper foundation of knowledge, clearly defined terms, rational concepts, and a quest for the truth.

BASIC CONCEPTS

The word *drug* needs a great deal of clarification. In medicine the word is used to refer to biologically active substances used in the treatment of disease. Thus, the concept would include such things as aspirin and antibiotics as well as the subjects of this chapter. What we are discussing here are the mind-altering drugs, or as they might also be called, psychoactive or consciousness-changing drugs. When any of these mind-altering drugs or substances are conceptualized as medicines, they are then reacted to psychologically in quite different ways than when thought of solely as drugs. Another basic dichotomy in our thinking is the conceptualization of such widely used and abused drugs as alcohol and nicotine as harmless beverages or cigarettes.

As I proposed several years ago, we might also refer to the mind-altering drugs as "pleasure-giving drugs," since the main reason these drugs are used is the expectation that they will bring pleasure in some form, even though this expectation often is not realized. The pleasure-giving concept also emphasizes one of the major reasons why users (excepting users of alcohol and tobacco, which are not seen as drugs) are condemned. Generally any socially disapproved mind-altering drug comes to be referred to as a narcotic or dope and the user as an addict. This mainly reflects police and newspaper practices as well as the false labeling, by criminal law, of such drugs as marijuana as "narcotics."

As the police have received some degree of education from physicians and social scientists, they have begun talking about marijuana as a "soft narcotic," which has about as much scientific meaning as a concept of "soft or mild pregnancy" would have. Rationality would be better served if we all began referring to these drugs by their individual names—alcohol, marijuana, LSD, etc. Particularly confusing with LSD-type drugs are the terms *hallucinogen* and *psychedelic* (mind-manifesting), both of which are unclear and misleading. The former emphasizes negative properties and the latter positive properties, neither of which is a uniform, consistent effect of this type of drug. This latter terminology also leads to the use of such words as *mild psychedelic* (often used in reference to marijuana) which in its characteristic effects throughout the world is no more (or less) psychedelic than alcohol. Psychedelic-type experiences can of course be obtained in association with a wide variety of nondrug experiences as well as with a number of the drugs under discussion here.

"Use" of a drug is another often much misunderstood concept. Almost all use (including abusive and addictive use) of socially approved and encouraged mind-altering drugs is usually equated with normal use, while conversely, almost any use of a socially disapproved or illegal drug is equated with abuse or addiction. Use can be one-time use, it can be occasional or intermittent use, or it can be regular use. Some regular use can be abusive use, and some abuse involves physical addiction. The drug families where this is possible include alcohol, sedatives, and narcotics (opium, morphine, heroin, meperidine, methadone, etc.).

Misuse or abuse of a drug should be thought of in terms of any use (usually chronic excessive use) which causes interference with the individual's social or vocational adjustment or health, or harms society. Habituation or psychological dependence can occur with any of the mind-altering drugs or with a variety of nondrug phenomena such as television. *Addiction* as a term should be used only in connection with physical dependence, which means, first, a development of tolerance by the body to a given drug and, second, a withdrawal illness or abstinence syndrome when the drug is discontinued or sharply reduced in dosage.

The use or abuse of any one mind-altering drug such as LSD can only be correctly understood by looking at the true and full context of mind-altering drug use. This would include alcohol (the most used and abused drug in this group, by both young and old); sedatives (barbiturates, chloral hydrate, Doriden®, meprobamate, and many others) ; stimulants (caffeine, nicotine, amphetamines, and cocaine), narcotics; marijuana (cannabis) ; miscellaneous substances such as glue, gasoline, and nutmeg, nitrous oxide and other gases; and the LSD family of drugs which includes mescaline (peyote), psilocybin, DMT, STP, yage, ibogaine and some sixty other known substances used in various parts of the world.

Perhaps the most important concept in the mind-altering drug world is that of the *drug effect,* an idea which is generally misunderstood and has led to a great deal of in-effective and dangerous social policy. What we call the drug effect and loosely attribute to some inherent property of the drug, is in reality a complex interaction between the pharmacological properties of the drug, the personality or character structure of the person consuming the drug (which is by far the major variable), and the social setting or con-text including cultural traditions, expectations, and the im-mediate environment. This is best illustrated by the most common group mind-altering drug experience in American society—the cocktail party. Here people consume similar amounts of the same drug within the same time period and yet behave in quite different ways, ranging from passivity to aggressiveness, and from impotency to lasciviousness.

Magical or propagandistic thinking about a given drug being directly and causally associated with violence or with religious mysticism is false or fraudulent as the case may be. The extreme and irrational polarities which sometimes domi-nate discussions of these drugs are best illustrated by using a political terminology—right-wing and left-wing positions. The right-wing point of view, usually expressed by narcotics police and some politicians, would have us believe that all people consuming LSD (or sometimes marijuana) will within minutes or hours of taking it be transformed into murderers, rapists, or lifelong inmates of mental hospitals. The left-wing point of view, usually expressed by psychedelic revolutionists, would have us believe that within hours of consuming LSD, all users would be transformed into fully self-actualized creative geniuses, living happily ever after.

Equally basic to understanding drug effects is the recognition that much bizarre, antisocial and criminal behavior occurs in our society without any association whatsoever with mind-altering drug use. The headlines we see often lead one to believe that all of our problems as a society are related to LSD use and, further, that if we simply arrest and imprison all users, all of our problems will be solved.

Other important variables in determining drug effects include the dosage, purity, method of administration, combinations with other drugs, preparation for the drug experience (cultural or individual), availability of supervision or help, etc. Thus, how the drug is used is more important than whether the drug itself is inherently beneficial or harmful, dangerous or harmless. Indiscriminate patterns of use, the use of unknown dosages or impure substances, and a lack of preparation and guidance are all conducive to a less than desirable experience or sometimes an unpleasant experience, or "bad trip."

Although logic and scientific method are considered by the educated segments of our population to be essential to the proper understanding of the world, the drug scene is almost totally bereft of such concepts. There is a notable absence of sampling techniques, use of control groups, statistical analysis, and elementary logical reasoning processes. Generalizations from some to all are quite common, as is extrapolation from pathological (hospitalized or imprisoned) examples to the general social pattern of use. Public organizations and legislative bodies often fail to hear any medical or scientific evidence before arriving at their far reaching conclusions, and they ordinarily receive all their information from individuals with little more than a high school education and who would not qualify as experts on the subject in any courtroom (this despite the fact that about two thirds of legislators are themselves lawyers who should understand expert qualifications). This situation is analagous to attempting to gain complete knowledge of farming or food processing from interviewing garbage collectors.

THE HISTORY OF USE OF THE MIND-ALTERING DRUGS

Alcohol has been used since at least the Old Stone Age one million years ago, and is extensively used and abused in most countries of the world; for it is essentially uncontrolled, overavailable, and strongly encouraged both by custom and by millions of dollars of advertising each year. In its short-term effects, alcohol, like the sedative drugs to which it is biologically equivalent, acts as a central nervous system depressant. It produces relaxation or sedation, sometimes euphoria and diminished inhibitions, and often (particularly with more than minimal doses) impairs judgment, coordination, and reaction time. The long-term effects include psychological dependence and sometimes physical dependence (addiction), or permanent damage to the brain, liver (cirrhosis), and peripheral nervous system. An estimated eighty million Americans use this drug, most of them regularly, and of this number some six million are alcoholics.

Other types of drug abuse associated with alcohol include highway deaths and injuries (50 percent of which are attributable to alcohol consumption), crime (alcohol is the only drug where scientific proof exists of its relationship to dangerous behavior), accidents and violence. This is emphasized by the fact that half the people in prisons committed their crimes in association with excessive alcohol consumption. And one third to one half of all arrests are for drunkeness. Other effects of alcoholism include mental illness (approximately 20 percent of the people in state hospitals are there for alcoholic brain damage), industrial absenteeism and job loss (costing many millions of dollars each year), family disruption, and so forth.

Anesthetic gases, sedatives and tranquilizers have short-term effects generally comparable to those described above for alcohol under the rubric of central nervous system depression. The gases are relatively unavailable although there is some use in this country of nitrous oxide present in aerosol cans. Sedatives and tranquilizers are widely available in various over-the-counter preparations (containing antihistaminics,, belladonna or scopolamine, and other ingredients) or acquired through physicians' prescriptions. These can frequently be refilled repeatedly, often in large quantities. Many millions of Americans use these drugs, and the number of abusers and sometimes addicts must range into hundreds of thousands, for enough barbiturates alone are produced each year in America to make more than thirty average doses for each man, woman and child. And about 20 per cent of all physicians' prescriptions are written for the several hundred preparations in this general category.

With the exception of alcohol, bromides are probably the oldest Western preparation in this family, but modern sedative history begins with the barbiturates, which came into use after 1912.

Although most of the use and abuse is among the middle and upper classes, there is also significant abuse among the young. The word *tranquilizer,* when properly used, refers to drugs such as the phenothiazines (Thorazine®, etc.), reserpine and Librium®, which are used medically in the treatment of anxiety or psychosis and which have little potential for psychological dependence or for abuse. These drugs, particularly Thorazine, are being widely used for the treatment of acute bad trips from LSD.

Stimulants as a group are the most widely used drugs in our society since both caffeine (in the form of coffee, tea and cola drinks) and nicotine (in the form of tobacco and cigarettes) are almost universally available and almost uncontrolled. Caffeine is used to relieve fatigue or sleepiness or to produce a "high," or euphoria. There is essentially no abuse although most users become psychologically dependent upon it. With nicotine we have a quite different situation, since its use is associated with enormous health problems, particularly cardiovascular disease, bronchitis, and lung cancer, as well as causing fires and air pollution. Despite this overwhelming abuse it is massively advertised and distributed without any meaningful controls. It is of interest historically that when tobacco and coffee were introduced into some Western societies, their use was looked upon in much the same way as the use of marijuana is now, and notably unsuccessful attempts were made to suppress and forbid this use.

More powerful in their central nervous system stimulating effects and their use to increase alertness, reduce fatigue, diminish appetite, prevent sleep, or produce euphoria are the amphetamines such as Dexedrine®, Benzedrine®, and methedrine (called meth or crystal), which have been in use since 1933. As with the barbituarates and other sedatives, the amphetamines and similar drugs such as Preludin® are used by millions of Americans, mostly on prescription from physicians. Abuse involving psychological dependence, the development of tolerance, and a toxic psychosis, is widespread both among middle and upper-class users and among youth who purchase it on the black market and frequently take it by injection rather than by mouth.

Narcotics—meaning opium, its derivitives, and their synthetic equivalents—are drugs used in medicine primarily for analgesia or relief of pain. Their history of use goes back about three thousand years for both pain and, presumably, pleasure. Morphine, the active principal of opium, was isolated in 1800 and heroin (diacetylmorphine) was produced in 1898. Also important in this context is the development of the hypodermic needle sometime in the 1840's. The development in the twentieth century of numerous synthetic narcotics, codeine, and a large number of narcotic-containing cough syrups assumes importance in the existing pattern of narcotic drug abuse. The first Federal Food and

Drug Law in the United States was passed in 1906, followed by the Harrison Narcotic Act of 1914. As has been the case throughout the world, the imposition of criminal sanctions against the use of a particular drug, in this case opium, has led to far more extensive use of more dangerous drugs by a wider segment of the population.

Illicit heroin users probably number around a hundred thousand, most of them from our large urban ghettos, minority group members, and products of deprivation and discrimination. A large but so far unmeasured number of middle and upper-class individuals are abusers of narcotics obtained from physicians' prescriptions, and abusive users of narcotic cough syrups certainly range into the tens of thousands. This drug family has a high overall potential for abuse, for physical dependence, and for psychological dependence. Their short-term effects include central nervous system depression and other effects similar to those of the alcohol-sedative group. Long-term effects of excessive use include weight loss, constipation and impotency or sterility, but fortunately all these are reversible when the drug is discontinued. The medical use of these drugs, particularly in the treatment of narcotic addicts, is greatly overcontrolled, particularly since there is essentially no relationship between the pattern of medical use and the widespread illicit traffic originating in such countries as Mexico, Thailand and Turkey.

Cannabis, or marijuana, has been used by mankind for about five thousand years, and the plant continues to be widely grown throughout the world and widely used, illicitly and licitly, in North, Central and South America, the West Indies, the Indian subcontinent, the Near East, and Africa. Pharmacologically it seems to have a mixed sedative-stimulant effect with the active principals being components of tetrahydrocannabinol. Cannabis, which comes from the dried leaves, tops or resin of the female hemp plant, is widely used in the indigenous medical systems of Asia and

Africa, was formerly used in the United States in a number of tonics and elixirs, and is reported in Western scientific literature as being a valuable antidepressant drug and antibiotic.

Its usual short-term effects include relaxation, euphoria, increased appetite, some alteration of time perception, and possible lessening of inhibitions. Although scientific research on humans has been suppressed by the Federal Bureau of Narcotics which controls the tax stamps necessary for legal possession of the drug, it seems reasonable to suspect that many of the aforementioned effects would be useful in medical practice, particularly the relaxing, appetite-stimulating, and euphoriant properties. The fact that the drug is available only in impure form with unknown dosage, the dearth of clinical research and the excessive penalties against its use make use unwise even though no physical dependence occurs and there are no physical effects even from chronic excessive use. Highly concentrated forms of the drug made from the resin and known by such names as hashish or charas sometimes produce hallucinatory experiences when used excessively.

Prior to the Federal Marijuana Tax Act of 1937 and the various similar state laws, there was moderate use of marijuana in various parts of the country by diverse social groups without real evidence of abuse. An extensive mythology was deliberately created and perpetuated by self-serving narcotics police and politicians, associating marijuana with violence, sexual immorality, narcotics, crime and, more recently, with LSD use. One of the criminogenic effects of the law was to drive the distribution underground where it came to overlap with heroin. In the last five years there has been a steady increase of marijuana use, mainly among youth and pervading all socioeconomic groups. The number of users are at least in the hundreds of thousands.

A wide range of miscellaneous substances are also used for mind-alteration, ranging from the inhalation of glue or gasoline fumes, to amyl nitrite, nutmeg and many others. It is particularly important to emphasize the ease of transfer or substitution of mind-altering substances which can occur when one becomes unavailable and also to illustrate the impossibility of controlling such complex phenomena simply by imposing criminal penalties against the user of a particular substance.

The *LSD-type* drugs, although in terms of public attention seem to be the newest form of mind-altering drugs, are actually one of the oldest, since the cactus peyote and its active principal ingredient, mescaline, have been used for at least two thousand years by the Aztecs and other Indian tribes of this continent. Spanish missionaries and administrators sought to suppress this use after the conquest of Mexico but were unsuccessful. Psilocybin and psilocin from a mushroom have been used for about four hundred years in various parts of Mexico as a part of religious rites in much the same way that peyote continues to be used by members of the Native American Church in the United States. Both of these drugs as well as LSD have also been used therapeutically, experimentally and illicitly.

The best known and most used presently of this group of drugs is d-lysergic acid diethylamide tartrate (LSD-25) which was synthesized in 1938 from ergot and accidentally discovered to have "hallucinogenic" properties in 1943. Many other synthetic and naturally occurring drugs with similar properties are also available. The first phase of LSD use mainly involved pharmacological and "psychotomimetic" studies. This was followed by experiments on creativity, treatment of character disorders, and religious mysticism. The present phase, involving widespread indiscriminate use mostly by young intellectually inclined people, stems from a combination of magical expectations which were created by the sensationalism of the mass media, the extremism of police and politicians, and the ready availability and ease of concealment of the drug. Regular users probably number no more than tens of thousands, but perhaps as many as one million people have used an LSD-type drug (usually LSD itself) in this country, not including the two hundred thousand members of the Native American Church who regularly use peyote.

The short-term effects include intense visual imagery and other sensory phenomena, euphoria or elation, and heightened intellectual functioning, all of these with LSD, lasting up to twelve hours with average doses. Acute panic reactions, precipitation of an already existing psychosis, recurrent psychedelic experiences, and accidental death or suicide occur in a minority of users in decreasing order of frequency. No physical damage to the body and no physical dependency occur. The present hysteria and legal penalties have greatly inhibited human scientific research with these drugs.

SOCIOLOGICAL ASPECTS

Mind-altering drug use and abuse is best understood as a barometer of a sick and corrupt society, as a reflection of underlying social storm. Americans live in a drug-ridden society where hundreds of millions of dollars are spent each year on advertising that encourages people to use alcohol, tobacco or other drugs every time they have a pain, a problem or trouble. Most adult Americans use between three and five mind-altering drugs each day including coffee, alcohol, nicotine, tranquilizers, sleeping pills and stimulants. Illegal drug use has become for the press and politicians a very convenient smoke screen in American society serving to obscure many more important social problems as well as obscuring much more serious drug problems such as alcoholism and the massive exporting of marijuana and heroin from Mexico into the United States. Such drug use also has important anti-intellectual and scapegoating functions directed against a significant segment of American youth and often artists, intellectuals and minority-group members.

An absurd cycle of hypocrisy and irrationality pervades

this field. This began with artificially created anecdotal stories about certain forms of drug usage and was followed by legislative testimony (by carefully selected cooperative police or medical politicians who usually have never dealt directly with drug use) and demagogic statements in political campaigns. Also involved is a strong element of puritanism (which does not concern itself with drugs such as alcohol), well defined by Mencken as "the haunting fear that someone, somewhere may be happy."

Throughout all this, the deep-seated roots of drug use are ignored. These include the curiosity and experimentation of the young, poverty and racial discrimination, boredom and monotony, alienation, the generation and credibility gaps, the criminogenic laws and their fanatical enforcement, the ready availability of the drugs, the sensationalism of the press, the peer-group pressures, advertising practices, etc. The American system of control of drugs socially disapproved at any given time has essentially been one of applying criminal penalties to users and continually increasing these penalties when the problem becomes worse, as it inevitably does. The system also includes the taking away of judicial discretion to grant probation or suspended sentences, restrictions on parole of convicted offenders and other similar measures which exceed in ferocity all other criminal laws except those against first degree murder. More drug police, more agencies, more jails and prisons, and so on, are created in a tragic illustration of Parkinson's law as bureaus have aggrandized their power and seek to justify their existence.

Because LSD use involves an odorless, colorless, tasteless substance of infinitesimal dosage, the laws against it are even less enforceable than those against alcohol between 1920 and 1933, although for different reasons. With LSD as with marijuana and narcotics, we have dual Federal and state laws involving overlapping and competing bureaucracies. One of the many inconsistencies and paradoxes in our drug laws is the inclusion of marijuana in the narcotic laws (meaning its possession is punished as a felony with prison sentences) while LSD, which everyone agrees has more dangerous effects, is under the "dangerous drug" laws (meaning possession is a misdemeanour punishable by either a fine or a shorter jail sentence). Another inconsistency is that in California, peyote (which is in the same family with LSD) is included under the narcotic laws, while LSD is placed in the dangerous drug laws.

Space does not permit an extensive discussion of the extreme penalties applied against those who possess these drugs and are caught or trapped with them, but it is important to point out that the Federal Drug Abuse Control amendments of 1965 (the basic Federal law covering stimulants, sedatives, and LSD-type drugs) *excludes possession* for one's own use as a criminal violation and thus sets a noteworthy example which should be emulated in other drug laws. Unfortunately the larger states, including California and New York, have superimposed traditional kinds of state legislation which include possession as well as sale or manufacture as criminal violations. But a vast number of other substances can be used for mind alteration, so if we continue the present system and are consistent in our illogic and irrationality, we will have to pass similar laws controlling even more of the environment. These will have to include regulation of gasoline and solvents (since their fumes are sometimes inhaled to get "high"—model glue has already been banned in this manner, for those under 21); *breathing* (carbon dioxide accumulation in the brain can lead to mind alteration), and *sleep* (sleep deprivation leads to mind alteration). Similarly we will need laws controlling the sensory environment, since sensory deprivation can produce mind alteration. Surely *1984* cannot be far away.

The consequences of our present American system of "control" are clear. In addition to the already mentioned increased use of more types of mind-altering drugs (many of them more dangerous) by more socioeconomic groups and occupations, we now have more involvement with organized crime, hypocrisy, corruption, disrespect of law and of police, spying, entrapment and informing. A large and increasing number of our youth are being labeled and stigmatized as criminals and deviants, are being taught crime in jails and prisons, and are driven from seeking help when they need it from professionals. A large number of police are diverted from pursuing real crime such as murder, rape and theft, all of which are sharply increasing. There has been a drastic reduction in scientific research and knowledge as a by-product of this system and those who seek needed reforms, rationality and objectivity are slandered, harassed and intimidated.

THE "SOLUTIONS"

It is usually better not to act at all than to rush into over-simplified pseudosolutions which make the problem—in this instance drug abuse—much worse. Hysteria, witch hunting, and irrationality must be avoided if progress is to be made. There are a variety of "controls" available to our society to deal with this or other complex social problems, and it is tragic that control has been seen only in terms of treating drug users as criminals and deviants. Much greater selectivity and individualization of approach is necessary. The use and abuse of mind-altering drugs should be recognized as a sociological and public health matter and sometimes problem, rather than a proper subject for the criminal law. Criminal penalties as a technique of control should be reserved for clearly antisocial behavior such as violence, theft and so forth, which can occur in association with or apart from drug use. Criminal penalties applied to drug problems should be reserved for illicit manufacture and distribution where this kind of control is clearly proven to be desirable. Such a reform would avoid the tragic effects on an already large and increasing number of youths and would eliminate the criminogenic effect of our present system. As part of this, such agencies as the Federal Bureau of Narcotics should be abolished, as was recommended by the President's Commission on Narcotic and Drug Abuse, and whatever specific kinds of enforcement powers are necessary should be incorporated into the Department of Justice nationally or general police work locally rather than delegated to the ineffective and often corrupt special narcotics squads. Use or possession for one's own use of an illegal drug should thus be excluded as a criminal offense as it is in the most recent Federal laws dealing with mind-altering drugs.

Great emphasis should be placed on public health education about these drugs, providing objective factual information, avoiding extreme and propagandistic statements which are rejected by most young people and actually increase drug use, and the properties of these drugs should be demythologized. Specific laws and regulations to implement them should be developed immediately to provide for the widest possible range of creative scientific research, particularly with marijuana and LSD-type drugs. Comprehensive outpatient treatment and rehabilitation programs for drug abusers, including all the types described above, such as San Francisco's Center for Special Problems (developed by the author), should be available in all our large cities. The present token emphasis on rehabilitation needs major augmentation along with changing our present concentration on prison hospitals and on narcotic addiction. Experts with extensive knowledge of the sociological, public health, and treatment aspects of drug abuse need to dominate policy development rather than calling upon police, medical politicians or administrators, and laboratory researchers whose experience with these problems is very limited or nonexistent.

Most importantly, we need to ask ourselves why so many people, young and old, need to turn to drugs, both legal and illegal, to find meaning or identity or happiness in our society. We need to understand and correct the social roots of the problem. There is also a need to increase our toleration for individuality and for differences in behavior, dress and beliefs. To the greatest extent possible, our society must be reformed and rebuilt to make a life a "mind-expanding" experience.

It is appropriate here to quote from a joint statement prepared by those of us on the program of the 1966 University of California LSD conference held in San Francisco. This statement said:

> We wish to indicate publicly our agreement on the necessity of avoiding hasty legislation with regard to these substances. We particularly wish to urge legislative bodies throughout the country to conduct thorough reviews of the subject prior to action and to enlist as wide a spectrum of expert advice and testimony as possible. The scientific, social, cultural and philosophical problems involved in the use of LSD and related substances are exceedingly complex. Legislative action which does not give adequate consideration to the complexity of these problems may defeat the very purpose for which it is intended and may create more serious difficulties. In cases where legislation has already been passed, it is recommended that the executive branches of the state and federal governments call conferences of experts from a broad range of fields, including pharmacology, psychology, psychiatry, criminology, anthropology, philosophy, theology, and the arts to provide guidelines for social control policies.

Bibliography

1. AMERICAN BAR ASSOCIATION AND THE AMERICAN MEDICAL ASSOCIATION JOINT COMMITTEE ON NARCOTIC DRUGS: *Drug Addiction: Crime or Disease?* Bloomington, Ind., Indiana, 1961.
2. ALPERT, R., *et al.*: *LSD.* New York, New Am. Lib. 1966.
3. *Ataractic and Hallucinogenic Drugs in Psychiatry.* Geneva, World Health Organization, 1958.
4. BECKER, H. S.: *Outsiders.* Glencoe, Ill., Free Press of Glencoe, Inc., 1963.

5. COHEN, A. K.: *Deviance and Control.* Englewood Cliffs, N.J., Prentice-Hall, 1966.
6. COHEN, S.: *The Beyond Within: The LSD Story.* New York, Atheneum, 1964.
7. DeROPP, R. S.: *Drugs and the Mind.* New York, Grove, 1957.
8. EBIN, D.: *The Drug Experience.* New York, Orion, 1961.
9. ELDRIDGE, W. B.: *Narcotics and the Law.* New York, N.Y.U., 1962.
10. FORT, J. (with BLUM, R., *et al.*) : *Utopiates.* New York, Atherton, 1964.
11. FORT, J.: Giver of delight or liberator of sin: Drug use and addiction in Asia. *United Nations Bulletin on Narcotics,* 1965.
12. FORT, J.: Narcotics: the international picture. *Calif. Youth Authority Quart., XIV,* 1961.
13. FORT, J.: Recommended future international action against abuses of alcohol and other drugs. *Brit. J. Addict.,* 1967.
14. FORT, J.: The problem of barbiturates in the U.S.A. *United Nations Bulletin on Narcotics,* 1964.
15. FORT, J.: Narcotics and the Law: A Review. *Calif. Law Rev., L,* 1962.
16. GOLDSTEIN, R.: *1 in 7: Drugs on Campus.* New York, Walker, 1966.
17. Hearings (of House of Representatives Appropriations Subcommittee) on Treasury Department, Federal Bureau of Narcotics, 90th Congress, 1967.
18. Hearings on taxation of marijuana, 75th Congress, 1937.
19. Hearings (of U.S. Senate Government Operations Subcommittee) on LSD, 89th Congress, 1966.
20. Hearings (of U. S. Senate Judiciary Subcommittee) on LSD and Marijuana Use on College Campuses, 89th Congress, 1966.
21. HUXLEY, A.: *Brave New World.* New York, Bantam. 1958.
22. LINDESMITH, A.: *The Addict and the Law.* Bloomington, Ind., Indiana, 1965.
23. MASTERS, R., and HOUSTON, J.: *The Varieties of Psychedelic Experience.* New York, Holt, 1966.
24. Peyote. *United Nations Bulletin on Narcotics, XI,* 1959.
25. *Proceedings of the White House Conference on Narcotic and Drug Abuse.* Washington, D. C., United States Government Printing Office, 1962.
26. SINCLAIR, A.: *Prohibition: The Era of Excess.* Boston, Little, 1962.
27. SOLOMON, D.: *LSD: The Consciousness-Expanding Drug.* New York, Putnam, 1964.
28. SOLOMON, D.: *The Marijuana Papers.* Indianapolis, Bobbs, 1966.

29. *Task Force Report: Narcotics and Drug Abuse, The President's Commission on Law Enforcement and Administration of Justice.* Washington, D.C., United States Government Printing Office, 1967.

30. TAYLOR, N.: *Narcotics: Nature's Dangerous Gifts.* Boulder, Colo., Delta, 1963.

31. *The Marijuana Problem in the City of New York.* Lancaster, Pa., Cattell, 1944.

32. *The President's Advisory Commission on Narcotic and Drug Addiction: Final Report.* Washington, D.C., United States Government Printing Office, 1963.

33. WIKLER, A.: *The Relation of Psychiatry to Pharmacology.* Baltimore, Williams & Wilkins, 1959.

Chapter II

A QUARTER CENTURY OF
RESEARCH WITH LSD

SIDNEY COHEN

INTRODUCTION

The first recorded reference to d-lysergic acid diethylamide tartrate (LSD) is A. Stoll and A. Hofmann's 1943 description of the synthesis of the drug and its oxytoxic effect on the rabbit's uterus (1). It was not until four years later that W.A. Stoll (2) reported the now classical instance of Dr. Albert Hofmann's accidental exposure and his subsequent deliberate self-experiment to establish the unusual psychic properties of LSD. The results of administering extremely small amounts (20 to 30 ug) were described as an acute exogenous intoxication. It is of interest to observe how the dosages have increased in later studies so that 1 to 2 ug/kg is administered therapeutically under certain conditions.

The diagnostic labels for the LSD state have also evolved during the intervening years. The toxic-confusional psychosis label was disputed by a group who considered the state to be a model psychosis, perhaps a mimicker of schizophrenia. Gerard suggested the name *psychotomimetic*. Still later, Osmond (3) offered the term *psychedelic* which withdrew it from the prejudicial category of psychoses and indicated that the state could go in a variety of directions, including positive, hyperphoric type of experiences, equated by some with chemical mystical states. At the present time, it can be suggested that the entire gamut of psychotic and nonpsychotic states may be witnessed by observers of large numbers of

LSD reactions: catatonic, paranoid or other varieties of schizophrenic syndromes, manic-depressive-like states, paranoia, toxic-confusional psychoses, somatization reactions, anxiety-ridden experiences, and still other mental states which have no psychiatric diagnostic equivalent.

Following the earliest studies, a gradual progression of the number of reports on LSD occurred until 1960. Since then about one hundred per year have been published in the scientific literature. Well over one thousand articles are available in English-language periodicals about the psychotomimetics of the lysergic acid series. During the past year a decline in the number of articles on LSD is evident.

PHARMACOLOGY

D-lysergic acid diethylamide is but one of an array of congeners. It is the most potent, but others have varying hallucinogenic capabilities, antiserotonin activity, and pyretogenic effects. No direct relationship seems to exist between the psychological properties of the group, their serotonin antagonism or their ability to raise body temperature. Of the lysergic acid group, ALD-52 (acetyl lysergic acid) approaches LSD in psychic activity. The levorotory isomer, l-LSD, is totally inactive as an hallucinogen. The necessary components of the molecule (see Fig. 1) appear to be 1) the indole group, 2) the substitution on the 4 position (in this respect it is similar to psilocybin and psilocin), 3) the
$$C-C-N\begin{smallmatrix}C\\\\C\end{smallmatrix}$$
attachment on the 3 position, and 4) the dextrorotary diethylamide substitution of the acid radical.

Ergot and a few other fungi contain lysergic acid, the inactive precursor of LSD. Some four species of the wild American morning glory seeds contain alkaloids which include isolysergic acid amide and lysergic acid amide. These agents are very weak psychotomimetics. The amino acids tyrosine and tryptophan are probable precursors to the lysergic acid compounds which occur in plants. LSD is synthesized

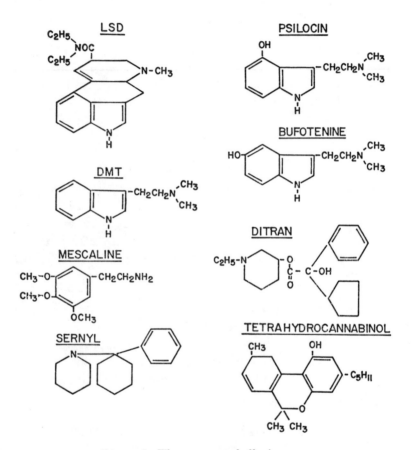

FIGURE 1. The common hallucinogens.

from lysergic acid and diethylamine. The tartrate is stable and readily soluble in water. It is an odorless, colorless and, if sufficiently dissolved, tasteless solution. LSD is readily absorbed from the gastrointestinal tract, mucous membranes, respiratory epithelium, and the abraded skin.

It has a decreasing latency period depending upon whether it is administered orally, subcutaneously, intramuscularly, intravenously, intraspinally or intrathecally. The delay in onset of subjective symptoms varies according to the amount and the route employed. The average latent period for 1 to 2 ug/kg orally is forty-five minutes (15 to 120 minutes). The effects of intravenous administration are noted within five minutes and the peak effects also occur more promptly. Intrathecal injection produces an almost instantaneous response. The duration of action is also dose-related to other factors such as individual sensitivity and deliberate, conscious efforts to abort or induce the state. If the drug has been swallowed, a gradual buildup of physiologic symptoms occurs. These may consist of numbness, a tingling of the extremities, feelings of chilliness, anorexia, nausea, vomiting (rarely), flushing, and dilation of the pupils. All of these except the mydriasis, partial cycloplegia, and other manifestations of central sympathetic dominance (quickening of the tendon reflexes, piloerection, hyperthermia, a mild hypertension, tachycardia and hyperglycemia) usually subside by the time the psychic symptoms appear.

In addition to the above-mentioned autonomic effects, LSD provokes a nonspecific stress response which is reflected by leucocytosis, eosinopenia, slight elevation of 17-ketosteroids and a moderate increase in 17-hydroxycorticoids. Plasma-free fatty acids are likewise increased. In animals exposed to LSD, increases in adrenal weights have been recorded.

The distribution of LSD in the body indicates that, although it readily crosses the blood-brain barrier, it is not preferentially concentrated in the brain. However, higher concentrations are found in the hypothalamus, limbic system, and the visual and auditory reflex centers than in the cortex and medulla. Recent studies reveal detectable amounts in the blood for periods extending throughout the period of drug activity, thereby invalidating the trigger theory which has been postulated when tracer studies on rats showed that is was essentially excreted within an hour. The half-life in man is calculated as 175 minutes. Excretion proceeds by way of 2-oxidation of LSD in the liver, an inactive metabolite, and the bulk of the substance is eliminated by the kidneys. No evidence exists for the binding of significant amounts of LSD to plasma proteins to account for the recurrences noted in a few individuals weeks or months following LSD usage. The prolongation of LSD activity beyond twenty-four to forty-eight hours also cannot be accounted for by postulating a retention of the chemical in the organism.

Tolerance to the effects of single daily doses of LSD is rapid and almost complete within four days. Koella *et al.* (4) has recently found that a cyclic escape of tolerance may occur in goats and other species including man. Abramson *et al.* (5) has noted a marked decrease in subjective symptoms when an average dose is given daily for three to four days. Tolerance to LSD is lost as quickly as it develops so that average amounts may be ingested at least twice weekly without impairment of drug activity. The tolerance effect can be avoided either by daily increases in the quantity of LSD used or by giving fractional doses of the drug every four to six hours. The manner by which rapid tolerance to LSD develops is unknown. Some of the speculations include 1) prevention of degradation of LSD into a more active metabolite, 2) a rapid enzymayic destruction of LSD into an inactive form, 3) phasic alterations of the blood-brain barrier, or 4) blocking of the receptor site at which LSD is active.

Cross-tolerance between LSD and other members of the

LSD series, including the nonhallucinogenic Brom-LSD, has been proven. Furthermore, cross-tolerance between LSD and mescaline, psilocin and dimethyltryptamine (DMT) is established. The anticholinergic hallucinogens, Ditran and Sernyl, do not induce cross-tolerance with LSD, indicating that this group may act on other pathways than do the indole and catechol amine hallucinogens.

Physical addiction, in the sense that withdrawal effects follow prolonged use of the drug, does not occur with LSD. Psychological dependency is now known since the agent has appeared on the black market. Periodic rather than continuous use is the customary pattern of consumption.

Stimulants such as amphetamine, methamphetamine and methylphenidate tend to potentiate and increase the euphoriant effect. Of course, marijuana and other hallucinogens will act synergistically when taken with LSD. Sedatives, tranquilizers and narcotics counteract the LSD effect. Although an occasional person will have a paradoxical effect from the administration of chlorpromazine (6), it is the antidote of choice if given in sufficient quantity. Barbiturates in hypnotic amounts are equally effective. The parenteral form of these antagonists are preferred when a rapid reversal of state is desired. Dosages of 500 to 1000 mg of sodium amobarbital intramuscularly or intravenously are required for a florid LSD excitement, and additional amounts may be required within a few hours.

One of the first of the subjective effects is a mobile, colorful patterning of the visual field with closed eyes. The more complex psychic phenomena to be described subsequently are noted later. Another hallmark of the LSD experience is the peculiar, phasic waxing and waning in intensity of the mental alterations. This may be so marked that the individual may believe that he is "back" only to find a few moments later that he is "way out." The undulations in the intensity of the state increase over the first two or three hours until a peak or plateau is reached. Then a gradual, undulating subsidence of the effects takes place until almost all manifestations of the LSD exposure are gone after eight to twelve hours. A few sensitive subjects given average amounts can detect some psychic alterations for as long as twenty-four hours. Very large doses may produce intense and substantial symptoms for forty-eight hours. The largest amount that has been given under medical supervision is about 1500 ug. Claims of ingestions up to 10,000 ug have been made by an occasional habitual user, but the accuracy of the amount and the quality of the substance is questionable.

The LD_{50} for man (lethal dose for 50 percent of a population) is unknown; an instance of death directly due to LSD poisoning has not yet been recorded. Whether nerve-cell changes occur from chronic or acute LSD usage in man is likewise not established. The lethal dose for 50 percent of mice, a species resistant to the drug, is 46 mg/kg. The LD_{50} for the rabbit is 0.3 mg/kg. If man metabolizes LSD like a rabbit, the calculated LD_{50} would be about 20 mg (or 20,000 ug). However, large-brained animals may be more sensitive to the lethal effects. An elephant convulsed and died in laryngospasm when 0.15 mg/kg was injected. For a 70 kg man, the LD_{50} may then be extrapolated at about 10 mg.

The ED_{50} (effective dose for 50 percent of a population) for LSD is thus much lower than the estimated LD_{50}. When death results in the course of an LSD experience, it is due to accident or suicide rather than its intrinsic toxicity. Since it is an intensely stressful psychological experience, it is possible that a person in marginal cardiac compensation may decompensate. The physical complications, except for a rare convulsion, are few. It is the psychological adverse effects which are impressive.

Sensitivity to a standard dose (100 ug) of LSD varies markedly. About 10 percent of a population will not observe any substantial subjective changes; the great majority will report definite psychic alterations. Women appear more sensitive that men. Schizophrenics and alcoholics are somewhat resistant to average amounts of the drug. Those who do not relish loss of their ego controls can successfully "fight off" ordinary doses. Body weight is not a reliable index of LSD sensitivity. Any dosage-response curve for the psychotomimetics would have to consider nonpersonality variables such as the security of the environment and the expectations of the subject and the observer. It is because of these nondrug variables that LSD has never found a place as a reliable psychodiagnostic test.

The question of human brain damage following prolonged, high dosage remains unresolved. Rats given 25 mg/kg in acute experiments evidenced vacuolization of nuclei, depletion and fragmentation of the Nissl substance, rarefaction, and degenerative cytoplasmic changes. Recently, the effects of various concentrations of LSD were studied in cultured human leucocytes which had been arrested in metaphase (7). Significant increases in chromosomal abnormalities, particularly in chromosome 1, were observed. The cytogentic investigation of one schizophrenic patient who had been treated with LSD over a four-year period (consisting of fifteen treatments in dosages ranging from 80-200 ug also revealed increased chromosomal breakage. Neither schizophrenia itself nor the use of tranquilizers has been shown to produce similar chromosomal alterations. The implication of this study is that large amounts of LSD taken frequently may interfere with cytogenetic architecture, but further work will have to be done to confirm this impression.

LSD has an effect upon the surface EEG reminiscent of the amphetamines. The typical pattern is one of low amplitude, fast wave activity similar to that seen in the awake, vigilant organism. Total electrical energy content and variability of the tracing are diminished. By use of a frequency analyzer the tracing is found to be altered after singles doses for days or weeks in mice. This alteration is nonspecific. Monroe (8), using depth electrodes, found that LSD activated seizure patterns in chronic schizophrenics in limbic system leads, and this paroxysmal activity coincided with an increase in psychotic behavior.

When single neurone leads were employed, Marrazzi (9) demonstrated synaptic inhibition in the transcallosal pathway. He also noted a disinhibiting effect on neurones in the visual tract. Pretreatment with chlorpromazine abolished the inhibition of inhibitory nerve cells.

The precise manner by which LSD exerts its manifold psychic effects is unknown. On the basis of the inhibitory action of specific nerve cell assemblies, certain assumptions might be made. Many of the inhibited tracts are known to act as inhibitors of direct sensory pathways, modulating or quenching their input. We (10) have some partial evidence that in certain individuals a drastic reduction of the sensory inflow will reduce or eliminate the LSD effect. One site of the drug activity appears to be on the altered coding of sensation, intensifying and magnifying certain sense data. Field-ground relationships are altered. The unmodulated sensory signals may overwhelm the evaluative function of the ego. They may fire across high-threshold pathways provoking synesthesias, the cross stimulation of one sense by another (seeing sound, etc.). They may maximally stimulate reward centers in the hypothalamus, evoking strong discharge of limbic system activity which is manifested as hyperemotionality. Depth electrode studies do reveal paroxysmal activity in the limbic system in the LSD-treated animals and in man. A failure of the quenching mechanism would result in enormously increased data content which could not be handled by the available data processing and data reduction facilities of the brain.

The neurochemical basis for the action of LSD likewise remains speculative. As noted, it is a strong serotonin antagonist; its mode of action was considered to be as a competitive inhibitor of serotonin in the central nervous system. However, other serotonin antagonists equally potent, which are capable of crossing the blood-brain barrier (Brom-LSD, for example), have little or no hallucinogenic effect. March-banks *et al.* (11) has found that LSD releases bound sero-tonin. In addition, it inactivates monamine oxidase and acetylcholinesterase. These effects would increase free nore-pinephrine, serotonin and acetylcholine levels in subcortical areas. Clearly, the biochemical mechanism of action is more complex than simple serotonin antagonism.

One of the peripheral results of LSD research has been a reawakening of interest in neurochemistry, both normal and pathological. If trace amounts of a substance could induce pronounced changes in perception, cognition, affect, and ego structure up to and including hallucinations, delusions and depersonalization, then the search for a chemical basis of mental activity could be rewarding. A biochemical substrate for schizophrenia would be worth researching. The serotonin hypothesis was generated as a result of Wolley's work with LSD. Aberrant norepinephrine metabolism must also inter-act in the disturbance of synaptic transmission and it, too, is markedly affected by LSD. Hoagland first demonstrated a decreased phosphate excertion in both untreated schizophre-nics and in normals given LSD. It now appears likely that a correlation between psychotic disorders and the excretion of biogenic amines exists.

In a study using rats, Ray (12) found that psychotogenic drugs produced a differential alteration in conditioning. Using animals trained to bar-press to receive food or avoid a shock, he found that LSD eliminated the conditioned response to food but not to shock. De Baran and Longo (13) likewise demonstrated that rabbits trained to respond to a buzzer which announced a food reward would lose this trained behavior after LSD. Of seven lysergic acid derivatives tested, the abolition of the conditioned response occurred in the hallucinogenic compounds, not in the nonhallucinogens. In most LSD studies using the conditioning model the conditioned response is lost, while the unconditioned response to pain is retained. This is also true of higher species including the baboon. We have data which indicate that conditioning and transfer of the conditioned response is more poorly accomplished in man. Some types of learning are therefore performed less well than under the nondrug condition.

The changes in psychophysiological test material during the LSD condition generally reveal a decrement of all items measured. Intelligence, psychomotor skills, reaction time, visual acuity, two-point discrimination, color thresholds, and all other measurements fall below baseline values. Attention span, abstract thinking, short-term memory, and mental arithmetic show a decrement. Some of these deficits result from loss of motivation to perform and difficulty in focussing on the task. The visual illusions (for example, the apparent movement of the printed word on the page) interfere with performance. Preoccupation with the sensory phenomena and a decrease in fine motor movements also worsen performance.

THE LSD STATE

In an evaluation of observations made from our first five-hundred subjects, the following overall comments can be made about the course of the LSD state. As mentioned, this is a highly variable condition, with the same subject under identical conditions sometimes undergoing exceedingly different kinds of responses. The variations are not random, however, and causative factors can usually be found to understand the varieties of LSD experiences. Some degree of reliability in predicting the nature of any single experience can be obtained by a thorough knowledge of the total situation. We have been able to alter our subject's emotional tone by behaving in a warm, friendly manner or by acting in a way which he interpreted as suspicious or nonsupporting.

LSD-induced alterations of personality function are dependent upon a number of nondrug variables in addition to being dose related. Needless to say, the underlying character structure is a significant feature of the resulting state. The expectations of the subject and those around him alter the experience by "programming" specific directions to a subject made exceedingly vulnerable to suggestion by attenuation or complete loss of his critical capacity. It is on this basis that the hypersuggestibility to verbal or nonverbal cues from the environment should be understood. The setting and feelings of security or insecurity will strongly influence the LSD state. When average doses of the drug are given to relatively stable individuals without prior indocrination, a wide range of reactions may be observed. The perceptual distortions and the changes in ego integrity produce a feeling of loss of mastery. This may be perceived as frightening if the situation is chaotic or the loss of control threatening. The "bum trip" can be the result of an encounter with an upsurge of personal problems or memories which had been concealed below the level of awareness. Bad experiences may also occur when ego controls cannot be relinquished or from fears of not coming back. The LSD state might be felt as blissful if the dissolution of the boundaries of the ego are interpreted as self-transcendence. The "good trip" is far from proof of an absence of repressed conflictual material. The personal unconscious can be evaded by a number of techniques.

Initially, the tendency is to try to "hold on," to resist the dissociation process. Eventually this becomes less possible, and the ego defenses which are brought into play are either exaggerated or overwhelmed.

Affect

Perhaps the first psychological indication that LSD has begun to act is a loosening of emotional inhibitions. Spontaneous laughter, sometimes tears, or smiling without particular cause indicate that the latent period is coming to a close. A relaxation of tensions is described not infrequently. Seemingly inappropriate and barely controllable laughter has dominated some experiences.

In general the mood tends to be euphoric and expansive, but labile mood swings are notable. The euphoria can mount to bliss, serenity, elation and joy. This aspect of the state is attractive to those who seek a chemical high. Extremely negative affectual responses are less common. These include tension, panic, fears of going mad or of an unknown, impending doom. A few subjects have remarked that their LSD encounter was marked by a complete absence of emotion, a sort of catatonic inability to feel anything. The feeling tone is reflected onto the other aspects of mental activity. Perceptual beauty is associated with pleasure and gaiety; flatness, drab colors, and fearful imagery with dysphoria.

Perception

The visual alterations dominate many LSD experiences. Remarkable metamorphoses of the percept are not unusual and are regarded as fascinating and unique. With eyes open, colors seem more brilliant and forms take on an added depth. The after-image is recognizably prolonged. Illusions, particularly the undulating movement of objects, are fairly regularly described. Close-in space is more strikingly altered than distant space. The significance of what is viewed may be enormously enhanced to the point where a smudge on the wall can become the key to the secret of existence. This overwhelming feeling of veridicality is another reflection of the failure of the critical function of the ego. Pseudo-hallucinations, projections of a concept onto the external world with a retention of the knowledge that it is unreal is sometimes reported as: "I can see a tall, thin man standing in the corner, but I know he really isn't there." True hallucinations are rather uncommon except in the higher dosage ranges.

With closed eyes, the subject attempts to describe a colorful, plastic pattern of ever-changing imagery. These chromatic geometries are called filigrees, wallpaper, modern art in motion, or kaleidoscopic visions. Later they become less symmetrical and more complex. Intricate stories are related of sequential events, some distant in time and space. They pass in review on the private screen behind the eyelids. When personal problems are dealt with, as in a therapeutic situation, this screen becomes the site of retrieved memories or symbols of the conflictual material. The intensity of the reaction increases when eyes are closed or covered. In a fearful reaction the subject may be unwilling to close his eyes.

Changes in what is heard are worthy of comment. Increase in the perception of sound, *hyperacusis,* is the most frequently remarked upon alteration. Those noises which are ordinarily ignored as unimportant and background enter into awareness—an interesting alteration of the auditory field-ground relationship. Auditory misperceptions are known, but auditory hallucinations are a rarity. Music may take on an enhanced meaning and intensity. Subjects have described becoming one with the musical composition, and some state that they never had really heard music before. Oddly enough, a number of the musicians tested related that they always heard music as they did under LSD. Some of them were more intrigued by the novel visual phenomena.

Tactile sensations are also modified. They are often described as more sensitive or more meaningful. Odors and tastes are altered, but ordinarily these are lesser changes.

The time sense undergoes substantial changes most frequently in the direction of a prolongation of subjective time. This phenomenon is observed with other central sympathetic stimulants such as the amphetamines and cocaine. "Time is standing still" or "A million things are happening between breaths" convey some idea of how radically internal time deviates from chronological time. This slowing down of personal time influences every aspect of the experience. The period of drug activity may seem endless; indeed, a few people have lost their temporal reference points and believed that they had been in the dissociation state for years and would never come back. Ecstatic states go on and on, and so do the horrendous ones.

Thinking

The drug-induced alterations of thought are manifold and complex. On small doses an acceleration of the thinking process is described; for some people the peripheral distractions may be eliminated and they are able to concentrate on minute cognitive areas. A flight of ideas and a copious, expanding flow of associative material may intervene, culminating in a hypomanic level of ideation. Thoughts become eidetic, that is projected as visualized images. They also interpenetrate and are modified by the ongoing feelings and sensations of the subject. This is a primordial thinking-feeling-sensing state probably similar to the mental activity of the infant.

Very often, and especially when high doses are employed, the thinking pattern is fantasy-laden with logical, rational mentation receding. These nonlogical, intuitive impressions are often accompanied by an innundating conviction of their validity. Unopposed by self-critical abilities, a thought may come to assume great power. Ideas that one can read minds and transmit messages to distant places can be overwhelming. One subject became frightened at his omnipotent thinking: "I might think myself dead, and if I did, I'd die." Ideas of reference—"Those people out there are talking about me"—are often expressed. Thoughts may acquire a dreamlike or nightmarish quality. Extreme notions of grandiosity or suspiciousness are entertained. Attempts to communicate content are only rarely successful and tend to destroy the thought sequence. A complete blocking of all mental activity for periods of time during the LSD episode is also mentioned. Recall for the LSD event is incomplete but better than dream recall. Confusion is rarely marked except at the higher dosage ranges and orientation is generally preserved.

Ego Function

Another striking effect of LSD is upon body image and self-concept. All sorts of feelings of physical alterations are recorded, from differences in size between the two halves of the body to changes in size comparable to those undergone by Alice in Wonderland. Duplication and triplication of the self are experienced. Feelings of strangeness about the surrounding space is common. The separation of external events from internal memories may become difficult or impossible. Likewise, the differentiation of the self from that which is outside might be lost as the ego boundaries dissolve. One's concept of oneself can undergo enhancement up to the heights of paranoid omnipotence; the opposite self-estimate is also a possibility. Denial and sublimation can be identified as modes of coping with the unusual internal and external changes. Regression with very dependent behavior is also seen.

Ordinarily, drives are in abeyance. Conventional beliefs and values are maintained by some who interpret the LSD state within the framework of their existing frame of reference. Others with less stable convictions are swept away by the enormity of the experience and undergo a complete revaluation with loss of their preexisting values.

Behavior

Behavioral patterns are usually predictable under experimental conditions. As a rule the subject is passive, sitting or lying quietly, saying little. His eyes may remain closed in order to increase the LSD effect. He may stare for hours at a single object. At times he requires urging to move, to go to the bathroom or to report the ongoing events. He may withdraw completely or continuously attempt a running account of the happenings. Task orientation is impaired. Activity can be stimulated by suggestion.

Other behaviors are possible, especially in the unstructured situation. Disrobing is mentioned from time to time. Hostile acting-out is known, especially when suspiciousness is prominent. When a complete loss of insight into the situation occurs, the subsequent behavior becomes unpredictable.

Ordinarily, individuals under the influence of LSD can pull themselves together and function according to the demands of the situation. Their judgment may remain impaired, and important decisions should be deferred until they have reviewed their decision in the sober state. Complex psychomotor tasks such as driving a car may be seriously impaired.

The Psychedelic Experience

Using the criteria suggested by Stace (14), LSD appears capable of mimicking the spontaneous transcendental experience. The elements of the chemical transcendent state are partly dose related, with the higher doses more likely to induce the visionary experience. The set and setting may be helpful although we have observed the state under doses as low as 75 ug in a drab hospital room in subjects unindocrinated to expect it. Panke (15) has done a controlled study on divinity students and obtained results which confirm this assumption. He administered either 30 mg psilocybin (equivalent to 300 ug LSD), or 200 mg nicotinic acid on a blind basis and found that those who received the psychedelic agent reported intense religious experiences as opposed to those who received the nicotinic acid.

The chemically induced state of transcendence includes all or some of the following elements:

1. There are complete feelings of unity with loss of self.

   This is a maximal loss of ego identity with accompanying

feelings of wonder, ecstasy or awe. It may be expressed as a turning point, a psychological death-rebirth experience.

2. One's sense of here and now is transcended. A feeling of timelessness and loss of spacial orientation is one aspect of the state. The condition seems to go on for a prolonged period although it may actually be momentary.

3. A sense of love and the sacredness of the event is apperceived.

4. Paradoxes are reconciled. Opposites cease to be polar and become an aspect of the whole.

5. The experience is considered indescribable, outside the realm of words, incommunicable, ineffable.

6. The rational, critical mind is in abeyance. It would be incompatible to be in a transcendent state and be able to examine it at the same time. Thought is essentially contentless.

7. The perceptual apparatus may be variously described as being involved with a "blinding white light" or "dazzling beauty." Only rarely is a visionary figure described in the psychedelic state although such a figure is "seen" more frequently in the spontaneous states.

Certainly further research is required into the neurophysiological basis for this unusual condition. From preliminary work with implanted electrodes in man, it may be speculated that maximal stimulation of the reward or pleasure centers in the midbrain may induce a similar ineffable, ecstatic, contentless, egoless experience.

To undergo such an experience, especially with chemical assistance, is far from a guarantee of an improved way of life either for oneself or in interacting with others. Even the more impressive spontaneous event, coming as it does "out of the blue," may change nothing. The psychedelic state could be an opportunity for a major reconstruction of one's life style, but it is no magical entree into the good life. Individuals have been seen who went through this tremendous psychedelic experience and emerged with overpowering messianic convictions. Others were so disappointed that nothing had changed that they were worse off than before their "enlightment." The psychedelic experience is a potent episode which may come prematurely in the course of a lifetime and be an unhinging factor.

The Psychotic Experience

As noted, the LSD exposure may mimic a transient episode of psychotic decompensation. This is the "freakout" or "bummer," in street parlance. It has only an indirect relationship to the prolonged psychotic break in that the experience characterized with a disorganizing, anxiety-ridden quality is somewhat more likely to lead to a prolonged major adverse reaction than a good trip.

The temporary LSD psychosis is characterized by a dysphoric-feeling tone of depression, dread and considerable fearfulness. The percept is likewise altered so that colors are in dark tones with dark green, brown and black predominating. Space appears flat and two-dimensional. People appear like caricatures or as ominous, threatening figures. Their faces assume a devilish or bestial character. One of the intolerable aspects of the situation is the fact that time does not pass, and the individual caught in a psychotic state may become convinced that he will remain in the state forever. Cognition is disorganized and repetitive thought sequences usually associated with hopelessness about the situation are expressed. One's self-concept is similarly altered. A feeling that one is tiny or hideously distorted may be mentioned. Guilt and worthlessness are often experienced. Delusions that one is about to die or disintegrate can be prominent. Absolute immobility, freezing, or running-away behavior may occur.

Some valuable aspects of the temporary LSD disorganization has been noted by Osmond (16). He believes it to be of value in the training of psychiatric personnel so that they may have an experience analagous to their patients' experiences. The distortions of space, time, thought and feeling can be known at first hand. A greater empathy with the difficulties under which the psychotic labors becomes more possible. It is a fine instrument for the study of the psychotic state. Osmond has administered LSD to an architect who designs psychiatric hospitals. The experience seems to have assisted the architect in developing a structure which diminishes the distortions of perspective and includes the psychotic's need for personal space.

LSD and Creativity

There are three questions to be asked about the interaction of LSD and creativity: 1) Does LSD enhance the creative process during the period of drug activity? 2) Does it produce prolonged improvement in originality of thought and execution? 3) Does the experience improve the appreciation for artistic and other types of creative expression?

A number of preliminary experiments have attempted to answer the first question. For example, artists have been given the drug, and their LSD productions were compared with their predrug drawings. As a rule these were judged to be worse because of the interference with motor function. In general, the paintings were more abstract, nonrepresentational and the brushwork more sweeping. Some of them were reminiscent of schizophrenic art. In a recent study, Harman (17) gave 200 mg mescaline (equivalent to 50 ug LSD) to a highly selected and motivated group of scientists, engineers and administrators who came to the experiment with a specific problem which they had been unable to solve. Acceptable solutions were achieved in a majority of instances. This indicates that focussing upon specific problems might be productive of some positive results in gifted people in a carefully structured setting. These were all subjects who had the potential for solving their problems stored within them, and the LSD acted to provide a novel way to view the problem and to retrieve the necessary data.

Whether a non-drug technique such as a brainstorming session might have been equally successful is unknown.

The second question has recently been the subject of a controlled study by the McGlothlins and me (18). We studied a group of seventy-two university graduate students before, two weeks after, and six months after three drug sessions. The best tests of creative thinking, flexibility of attitudes, anxiety levels and personality change were used. The experimental group of twenty-four men received 200 ug LSD on three occasions. One control group received 25 ug LSD and a second, 20 mg dextroamphetamine. The drugs were given in an optimal environment in the hope that the best possible experience would be achieved. The test results indicated no objective change in the direction of increased creativity; more members of the high-dose LSD group mentioned an increased subjective feeling of creative enhancement than the control group. This divergence between subjective impression of change and the inability to demonstrate a change objectively is noted in many areas of LSD activity. Enormous insights are frequently not followed by modified patterns of behaivor. Although the feeling of vast internal alterations may be sufficient to induce new ways of living in a few instances, most LSD conversions tend to be short lived unless reinforced with subsequent reeducation.

Our LSD subjects and those in other studies reported an increase in interest in and appreciation of esthetic activities. It seems likely that some people will come away from the LSD state with new or renewed esthetic interests.

CONCLUSION

With the current curtailment of research efforts involving the hallucinogens, many of the important questions still unanswered may remain so for decades. Questions such as the nature of the chemical action of a drug like LSD, how it produces its remarkable psychic changes, the incidence of side effects, the issue of neurotoxicity, its psychotherapeutic potential—all these and many other vital matters seem destined to be studied at a decelerated pace until the current sociological problems are resolved.

As with hypnosis, discredited when it fell into the hands of vaudeville performers and parlor hypnotists, LSD research may also decline for many years. During the past two decades the experimental study of the hypnotic state has been resumed after a hiatus of over half a century. The fate of future investigations into the various LSD states is not predictable.

Bibliography

1. STOLL, A., and HOFMANN, A.: Partialsynthese von Alkaloiden vom Typus des Ergobasins. *Helv Chim Acta, 26*:944, 1943.
2. STOLL, W. A.: Lysergsaure-diathy-amid, ein Phantasticum aus der Mutterkorngruppe. *Schweiz Arch Neurol Psychiat, 60*:279, 1947.
3. OSMOND, H.: A review of the clinical effects of psychotomimetic agents. *Ann NY Acad Sci, 66*:418, 1957.
4. KOELLA, W. P., and BERGEN, J. R.: Cyclic Response to Repeated LSD Administration. Presented at the annual meeting of the American College of Psychopharmacology, San Juan, Puerto Rico, Jan., 1967.
5. Abramson, H.A.; Jarvick, M.E.; Gorin, M.H., and Hirsh, M.W.: LSD: XVII tolerance and its relationship to a theory of psychosis. *J Psychol, 41*:81, 1956.
6. Schwarz, C. J.: Personal communication.
7. Cohen, M. M., and Marinello, M. J.: Chromosomal damage in human leukocytes induced by lysergic acid diethylamide. *Science, 155*:1417, 1967.
8. Monroe, R. R.; Heath, G.W.; Mickle, W. A., and Llewellyn, R.C.: Correlation of rhinencephalicelectrogram and behavior: A study on humans under the influence of LSD and mescaline. *Electroencep Clin Neurophysiol, 9*:623, 1957.
9. Marrazzi, A. S.: Synaptic and behavioral correlates of psychotherapeutic and related drug actions. *Ann NY Acad Sci, 96*:211, 1962.
10. Cohen, S., and Edwards, A. E.: The interaction of LSD and sensory deprivation: Physiological considerations. In Wortis, J., (Ed.): *Recent Advances in Biological Psychiatry.* New York, Plenum Press, 1964, vol VI, p. 139.

11. Marchbanks, R. M., Rosenblatt, F., and O'Brien, R. D.: Serotonin binding to nerve ending particles of the rat brain and its inhibition by LSD. *Science, 144*:1135, 1964.

12. Ray, O. S.: Effect of psychotogens on approach and avoidance behavior. *Int J Neuropsychiat, 1*:98, 1965.

13. De Baran, L., and Longo, V. G.: Instrumental reward discrimination in rabbits. EEG and behavioral effects in a series of lysergic acid derivatives. In Mikelson, M. Y., and Longo, V. G. (Eds.): *Pharmacology of Conditioning, Learning, and Retention.* New York, Macmillan, 1965, vol. I, p. 319.

14. Stace, W. T.: *Philosophy and Mysticism.* Philadelphia, Lippincott, 1960.

15. Panke, W. N.: Drugs and Mysticism: An Analysis of the Relationship Between Psychedelic Drugs and the Mystical Consciousness. Doctoral Dissertation, Harvard University, Cambridge, Mass. 1963.

16. Osmond, H.: Some Problems in the Use of LSD-25 in the Treatment of Alcoholism. Read at the Second Conference on the Use of LSD in Psychotherapy, Amityville, L.I., N.Y. May 8-10, 1965.

17. Harman, W. W.; McKim, R. H.; Mogar, R. E.; Fadiman, J., and Stolaroff, M. J.: Psychedelic agents in creative problem-solving: A pilot study. *Psychol Rep, 19*:211, 1966. *Monograph Suppl.,* 2-V19.

18. McGlothlin, W. H.; Cohen, S., and McGlothlin, M. S.: Long Lasting Effects of LSD on Normals. Read at the Fifth Annual Meeting of the American College of Neuropharmacology, San Juan, Puerto Rico, Dec. 7-9, 1966.

Chapter III

THE VALUE OF LSD IN PSYCHOTHERAPY

KEITH S. DITMAN
(In collaboration with Thelma Moss, Ph.D.*)

Sensationalism and emotionalism have so influenced the opinion of LSD among the general public (and scientists too) that serious investigation of all of the hallucinogens has been severely threatened. The mélange of newspaper and magazine articles, television interviews, and movies has often been irresponsible and created more problems than it has solved. Their effect all too often has been to increase the incidence of drug abuse, alarm but not always correctly inform the public, and help annihilate the legitimate study of LSD and other psychedelic drugs. A powerful piece of work has been done in obscuring the large body of scientific data which has been steadily accumulating in the professional journals for more than twenty years. This literature contains literally thousands of articles which present considerable pertinent information concerning the pharmacological, clinical, and therapeutic effects of lysergic acid diethylamide-25 when used in a supervised medical setting by qualified psychiatrists and psychologists who are familiar with the many and extraordinary effects of the drug.

Some of this early literature consists of anecdotal, personal experiences with the drug by highly gifted, nonmedical persons such as Aldous Huxley (1) and Allan Watts (2).

---
*Assistant Professor of Medical Psychology, UCLA Center for the Health Sciences, Los Angeles, California.

These accounts related chiefly the transcendental, mystical effects of the LSD experience. This information, suggesting potentially valuable avenues for research in psychiatry and religion, has been misused by the present lunatic fringe of LSD enthusiasts. Before an adequate understanding of the modes of action and effects are obtained, the "new religion" exponents such as Leary and Alpert and the hippies have come up with the injunction to "turn on, tune in, and drop out" under the influence of homemade LSD manufactured by questionable chemists and sold by black marketeers.

Concurrent with those early literary works, serious investigators like Sandison (3, 4), Abramson (5, 6, 7), Frederking (12) and Savage (13, 14) were exploring the use of LSD as an aid to psychotherapy. In fact, a considerable number of articles (well over 500) were published before 1960, in which claims were made that psychiatric patients suffering from a wide variety of mental and emotional disorders—including alcoholism, psychosis, suicidal depression, neuroses, homosexuality, frigidity and other sexual problems, as well as phobias and compulsions—were substantially benefitted from therapy with LSD. Subsequently, scientists from seventeen countries (including Czechoslovakia, Poland, South Africa, and Australia) have reported results with LSD as a therapeutic agent; results ranged from "no improvement" to "cured," usually with the largest percentage in the "improved" category. The range of illnesses treated now extends to autistic children—Bender (15), Abramson (10, 11), Simmons (16); alcoholics— Van Dusen (17), O'Reilly (18), Smith (19), Chwelos (20), Ditman (21, 22); paranoid schizophrenics—Grof (23); and psychopaths.

Admittedly, the majority of these studies are anecdotal case histories and clinical studies with no or inadequate control groups against which to compare results. And many of the authors made extravagant claims for LSD treatment— an all-too-familiar phenomenon with new and seemingly revolutionary methods of psychotherapy. Also, some of the investigators were not suited to render a responsible evaluation of a unique psychotherapeutic tool. However, these are problems in evaluating any psychiatric treatment; they are not limited to LSD therapy. One has only to remember the conflicting claims made for psychoanalysis in the early days of that movement; of electroshock therapy for depressives; of glutamic acid for mental retardates; hypnosis for the curing of symptoms such as stuttering, enuresis and the like; and more recently for the antipsychotic, antidepressive and antianxiety drugs to prevent or cure mental illness; and the behavior therapies such as Wolpe's (24) "reciprocal inhibition" based on learning theory. Although such extravagant claims gave way in time to a more cautious view of the therapies concerned, it nevertheless can be argued that, after the first glow of enthusiasm which seemed almost messianic, several of the aforesaid therapeutic techniques have proved effective in otherwise intractible cases. In fact, it becomes increasingly apparent that certain patients who do not respond to a specific form of treatment by one doctor will respond to a different form of treatment with another doctor. One must always be cognizant of the ever-present placebo response in which expectancy of the patient, the *belief* of both patient and therapist in the treatment, and the setting are so important in determining outcome.

Whether LSD therapy will eventually prove slightly, moderately, or vastly successful as a treatment modality for any psychiatric disorder remains to be evaluated. Meanwhile it certainly should not be denied further exploration provided that the exploration is done in well-designed studies under proper medical supervision, with all the necessary precautions observed. Surely fresh approaches to the treatment of psychiatric patients are sorely needed. What psychiatrist can claim infallibility in his methods? Indeed, what psychiatrist can prove that he is equipped to deal successfully with

the chronic alcoholic or the neurotic using the methods
available today?

Let us examine how LSD has been used as a therapeutic
agent. Immediately it becomes clear that the benefiicial
results claimed for the drug may not be solely due to its
pharmacological action. In fact, at present we do not know
for certain what the action of LSD is in the body, despite
literally hundreds of studies which have probed into the
problems of its possible sites of action in blood, brain,
neurons, organs and cells.

More definite information is available about the psychological effects of LSD *when used in psychotherapy by qualified psychiatrists.* Repeatedly in the literature of LSD therapy
(given in small doses ranging from 50 to 200 ug at each of
several sessions) we find descriptions of patients who undergo catharsis and abreaction, through the reliving of early
infantile or childhood traumata. The bulk of these studies
have been reported by therapists with a psychoanalytic orientation, whether Freudian, neo-Freudian or even Jungian
[Abramson (5, 6, 7), Martin (25), Buckman (26), Sandison (3, 4), van Rhijn (27, 28), Grof (23)]. It has been
suggested (whether consciously or unconsciously) that these
psychiatrists have somehow directed their patients toward
early experiences in order to follow the classical therapeutic,
regressive model. And it has also been debated whether
these early, repressed incidents which are recovered in the
LSD experience are in fact truly, realities relived; or whether
they are fantasies evoked for the sake of the therapist through
the disinhibiting effects of the LSD experience.

In some instances it has been possible to verify the recovered traumatic episodes by direct inquiry of parents and
other key figures concerning the specific events. Frederking
(12) reports the case history of a young man who had
always been impotent. Under the influence of LSD, he re-
gressed to "a small, helpless child subject to titillation of the
navel and genitalia and other kinds of trauma. (Later) upon

questioning his mother it was found that for several months, in the first half of his second year, he had had much to suffer at the hands of a nurse." Another case history of a frigid woman (29) describes an LSD experience in which the patient suddenly felt compelled to fling her arms across her body "as if in a straitjacket," and she was then unable to move her arms. During this experience she seemed to feel herself to be a very small child, in a crib, whose arms had been tied down so that she was unable to "scratch herself" around the genital area. The patient believed this was a punishment for attempted masturbation. But in the interval between LSD sessions, a rash developed around her genitals which her doctor was unable to diagnose. Subsequently she learned from her mother that at the age of two she had had chicken pox, and had been tied down so that she would not be able to "scratch herself." Grof (23) reports a case of a neurotic woman who under LSD relived an early sexual assault by her stepfather in the bathroom of her home—features of which stood out vividly in her mind and were subsequently verified. Sandison (4) describes still another early childhood sexual assault by a man in a forest on a young girl who later became the victim of a compulsion to wash herself, her clothes and her children's clothes incessantly. This episode was also proved to have happened in a forest which was almost identical to the one described by the patient under LSD. Perhaps the most startling abreaction is the one reported by a mature woman, under LSD (30), who felt herself to become tiny, "a helpless baby . . . feeling very cold and hungry . . . seeing nothing but white, white tile . . . ." Several weeks after this LSD experience, the woman learned from her mother, to her complete amazement, that she had been placed in an incubator for several days directly after her birth—a fact which she had not consciously known for all of her life.

In contrast to these LSD abreactions, which presumably have been verified, are those "abreactions" which seem to reflect *symbolic* reliving—a psychic reality rather than a specific episode from early life. One patient described by Arendsen-Hein (30) reported he felt himself "crushed in the womb, and not allowed to emerge because he was a boy instead of the desired girl his father wanted." Although this episode (experienced with excruciating pain and intensity) can hardly be considered an actual experience—except by some psychedelic panegyrists—it nevertheless embodies the patient's primary conflict: his attraction to homosexuality, which had become so powerful that it was destroying his marriage. Other instances of symbolic reliving are quoted by Sandison (3, 4) who gives as one example this patient's actual written words, after the experience, in which she describes "serpents' faces all over the wall . . . then I saw myself as a fat, potbellied snake—slithering gaily away to destruction. I felt horrified and thought, 'Whose destruction?' I then realized it was my own." And still another instance is quoted by Newland (29) in which the patient saw herself as a baby in a crib, terrified by a loudly ticking alarm clock, and by turning away from it, she then saw her mother and father engaged in the primal scene. This episode could not be verified and was assumed by the patient to be a symbolic representation of her horror in relation to adult sexuality.

Whether such vivid upsurges of psychic material are based on actual events or, rather, are symbolic representations of conflict-laden areas does not seem of much relevance when, as a result of such LSD-induced fantasies, the patient achieves greater insight and ability to resolve the problems which have been crippling his day-to-day living. Surely, it should not be necessary to say that insight and better ability to cope with the problems of reality are considered the twin goals of traditional psychotherapy, whether psychoanalytically oriented or not.

Thus far the therapy here explored with LSD has been defined by Leuner (31) as *psycholytic* rather than *psy-*

chedelic therapy. The difference, according to Leuner, is that psycholytic therapy describes a continuing series of LSD sessions with a therapist, in which over a period of months the basic conflicts and symptoms are uncovered through ventilation, catharsis and abreaction. There is activation and deepening of the psychoanalytic process. Such a course of treatment, this author declares, ranges from fifteen through sixty sessions, the average in his experience being thirty-eight sessions for each patient. Grof (32) also describes this kind of psycholytic therapy in his monograph, which reports on case histories of eighty patients treated with LSD in the Neuropsychiatric Institute at Prague, Czechoslovakia, with extremely beneficial results.

Psychedelic therapy, a different approach to LSD therapy, has been developed concomitantly. In this form of LSD therapy a single massive dosage (200 ug up to 1500 ug) is given to the patient in one protracted session in order to achieve the "rebirth" or "transcendental" conversion experience. The aim of such therapy is that the patient achieve the rebirth of his "self," and thus be cleansed and transformed, apparently in much the same manner that Saul (afterwards St. Paul) experienced his transformation on the road to Damascus. Many reports have appeared describing this type of psychedelic therapy with LSD, sometimes combined with carbon dioxide or mescaline or psilocybin [Mogar and Savage (33), Chwelos (20) and others]. In particular, this type of therapy has been claimed to be extremely helpful with chronic alcoholics who have not responded to any other form of treatment [Chwelos (20), Smith (19), O'Reilly (18), Van Dusen *et al.* (17)] with results ranging from 50 to 90 percent abstinence in patients who have been followed up from two months to one year after therapy. The aim of this kind of LSD experience is *not* to regress, to relive trauma, or to experience abreaction. Rather, the aim is to create in the patient a feeling of a new awareness of self, aesthetic appreciation and even religious ecstasy, in which the patient has a new outlook, feels cleansed and reborn, without the need for the crutches he has been using to sustain himself—crutches such as alcohol or other neurotic patterns of defense such as phobias, frigidity, depression, or psychosomatic illnesses. Again, claims for this kind of therapy have at times been extravagant, and as yet there have been inadequate controls or follow-ups to determine the length of time such "improvement" persists.

This "transcendental" experience under LSD has been the experience most publicized and most usually attempted by those that abuse the drug by taking it in nonmedical settings. This type of abuse has probably heightened the development of the hippie movement (which advocates tribal living, inner knowledge, and many of whom follow the dictum of "turn on, tune in, and drop out"). This mass youth movement with its multidrug abuse (a worldwide phenomenon reported in such diverse countries as Japan, Czechoslovakia, Sweden, and Argentina) has done much to make LSD and other psychedelic drugs objects of controversy and concern.

Several therapists have reported that a transcendental experience occurs in the course of their more traditional, psychoanalytically oriented therapies and is of occasional value in establishing a sense of belonging and personal worth which has long been missing in the particular patient. Some therapists caution that this mystical experience can be only a transitory phenomenon unless the basic conflicts are worked through and resolved. This is a controversy which is still being fought in much the same manner that the classical psychoanalyst argues with the existential therapist who does not concern himself with past events, but deals only in the here-and-now. Is the rebirth temporary, or longlasting? There seems to be no answer yet to this 2000-year-old question of the "faith cures"—whether at Galilee, Lourdes or in modern pharmacologic-religio-mystic experiences.

In sharp contrast to the therapeutic experience of LSD are the clarion cries of those opponents to the use of the drug who claim it causes, at the least, confusion; more typically, brain damage, suicide, murder and a variety of psychiatric illnesses, including psychosis. Amid these outcries are cogent warnings about the use of LSD. Among them are such reports as those by Ditman and Cohen (34) ; Ungerleider and Fisher (35) ; and Grinker (36). These authors have pointed out some disastrous results consequent to LSD ingestion: temporary psychosis, acute panic reactions, and severe bodily injury. These results cannot be denied.

But again, reports such as these are anecdotal case histories and are not from carefully controlled studies from which one could conclude that the disasters are attributable solely to LSD usage. There well may be other important variables which contribute or cause these dire consequences. Some of these variables are discussed below.

Other Drugs

Since LSD is being made illicitly in several states and countries, it is unknown what impurities and what amounts of LSD are in the so-called LSD purchased on the black market. Also, it is certainly common practice among drug abusers to combine LSD with a wide variety of other drugs such as marijuana, hasheesh, amphetamines and barbiturates. These other drugs are used to intensify and prolong the experience and to insure against a bad trip. Can it, then, be claimed that LSD is the *sole* cause for the calamities which have occurred among the drug abusers?

Nontherapeutic Settings

The heated and repeated statement that LSD is a harmful and dangerous drug which should be banned legally is a claim referring usually (though often not so explicitly stated) to the effects of the drug when taken in a nonsupervised and nonmedical setting. However, the majority of tragic instances resulting from LSD trips have occurred in an unsupervised, nonmedical setting—often among groups of people gathered together for greater gaiety and sensory enjoyment than can be offered by alcohol or other more orthodox intoxicants. Actually, the bad trip with its accoutrements of horrifying thoughts and perceptions, paranoia and panic may be much more the rule than the exception in nonmedical settings when compared with the therapeutic setting where LSD is used to elucidate distressing symptoms and behavioral disorders. But even in the therapeutic setting Grof (23, 32), for example, reports that several of his patients who were given psycholytic therapy responded to an LSD session by succumbing to a psychotic episode. Instead of terminating the therapy, Grof permitted the psychosis and then after only a day or two respite gave the patients another LSD session. His rationale was that the psychosis resulted from an overwhelming amount of repressed material with which the patient had been unable to cope, and the additional LSD session conducted by the same therapist then enabled the patient to become more familiar with the dreaded historical material, so that he could come to terms with it and assimilate the knowledge. After which, Grof claims, the therapy proceeded beneficently, with "some" or "considerable" improvement over a lengthy follow-up period. Although, so far as we know, such a drastic form of LSD therapy has not been used by other psychiatrists, there are numerous cases in which agony (either physical or mental) has been described by both doctors and patients. On some occasions the patients themselves achieved insights into the reason for their nightmare-fantasies during the same LSD session; on other occasions such material has been interpreted to the patient with constructive results by the therapist. More frequently, the process of insight and integration is described as a process which occurs over several sessions, both under the drug and in interviews between drug sessions.

Some therapists feel that the sudden shattering of defenses under LSD is too powerful an experience for some patients;

and for those cases Ling and Buckman (37), for example, have devised a therapy which, in addition to oral LSD, includes intramuscular injection of methylphenidate (Ritalin®) to lessen anxiety and give the patient more tolerance for the stressful, repressed material which explodes into awareness. Leuner (31) also adopted this method with some of his patients, but now cautions that the use of methylphenidate sometimes produces a "shallow ecstasy" so gratifying to the patient that he will cease all work on his problems and simply wait impatiently for the "bliss" which follows immediately upon injection. Another article by Ditman *et al.* (38) cautions against the use of methylphenidate except under the strictest medical supervision, because of that drug's highly addictive properties when taken intravenously or intramuscularly.

The panic and anxiety engendered by a bad LSD trip, then, may possibly be of therapeutic value when administered in a medical setting by competent therapists who will use those feelings as guideposts to lead to the heart of the emotional problems. Without such supervision, it is not at all surprising that LSD can provoke such violent emotions as panic, aggression, and suicidal impulses. In support of this view, a recent study by Ditman *et al.* (39) reports that those persons who have had to be hospitalized or had become psychiatric outpatients after LSD usage have retrospectively described their LSD experiences (by means of a 156-item Card Sort, on a five-point rating scale) as being far more anxiety-arousing—with significantly more fears of insanity, thoughts of death and even suicidal ideation and "disgusting sexual ideas" which came to the fore—than a comparable group of LSD takers who did not have to be hospitalized or treated as a result of their drug usage. It might then be conjectured that in a responsible medical setting the disturbing thoughts and accompanying anxiety or panic released by LSD can be used to therapeutic advantage, whereas in a nonmedical, thrill-seeking atmosphere, such material can precipitate prolonged anxiety, depression, obsessional states and even acute and chronic psychotic episodes.

By way of analogy, no one will deny that morphine, when abused in a nonmedical setting, is a dangerously addictive drug; yet when taken for the relief of intractible pain under medical supervision it has been quite a safe drug and a god-send to innumerable patients.

To plead for the wholesale banishment of LSD from medical use and scientific investigation because of its disastrous effects when taken in an irresponsible way seems an unwarranted and irresponsible act against the public interest. Such a precedent has already been established with a far milder psychedelic drug—marijuana—with the result that scientists know little of this drug's action, while an ever increasing number of the hippies and teen-agers abuse it for illicit pleasures. It is urgently pleaded that more careful consideration be given to legislation and its effects before we add further to the problem by hindering understanding and research and by subjecting the curious or the ill seeking some help to senseless punishment and stress.

Physiological Dangers

One of the most serious arguments against the use of LSD is that it may be causing brain or chromosomal damage. As of this writing, these claims have been based on a few studies (40, 41) with small numbers of experimental subjects being used. Currently, much more extensive investigations are being conducted at several medical centers. One study already completed, with nine LSD users contributing their blood for detection of chromosomal damage, reported (41) that it had been extremely difficult to find subjects who had taken *only* LSD. Of the nine subjects studied, the majority claimed to have taken many other drugs, including marijuana, hasheesh, peyote, stimulants, tranquillizers and sedatives. Given such circumstances, can one conclude that it is the LSD alone which is causing the chromosomal damage? The authors wonder if it is.

However, the possibility remains that LSD may cause either temporary or permanent damage to the chromosomes of the white blood cells and perhaps other parts of the body. Should the damage to other parts of the body be permanent, then—as has been warned—there may be a repetition of the tragedies which overtook the victims of mothers who had been given thalidomide while pregnant. As of this writing, there have been no mutants reported born to human LSD takers (and there have been many children born to such parents). Such reports have been made in studies on rats, however (42). In humans it may be that the effects of the drug will not become apparent until many years after birth, as with certain diseases and other drugs. Therefore, until it is definitely determined whether or not LSD does in fact produce chromosomal or brain damage, and the meaning of such possible damage is thoroughly understood, the authors feel strongly that further clinical usage of LSD in humans be limited to those conditions where there are indications of benefit and where the severity of the disease or prognosis countermands the possible risks. Also, such psychedelic drugs as mescaline and psilocybin can produce an experience similar to if not identical with that produced by LSD, and these drugs have not been reported to cause organic damage. Consequently, their substitution for LSD in psychotherapy research and other clinical work with humans would seem to be indicated.

Lastly, it should be emphasized that laws which dissuade qualified investigators from doing research with unique drugs like LSD can only be deplored. The psychedelic drugs do offer new frontiers for the exploration of brain mechanisms, the causes and treatment of mental illness—as well as areas of research involving the creative process, religion and possibly parapsychology.

Bibliography

1. HUXLEY, A.: *The Doors of Perception.* New York, Harper, 1954.
2. WATTS, A.: *The Joyous Cosmology.* New York, Pantheon, 1962.
3. SANDISON, R.A.; SPENCER, A.M., and WHITELAW, J.D.A.: The therapeutic value of lysergic acid diethylamide. *J Ment Sci, 100*:49, 1954.
4. SANDISON, R.A., and WHITELAM, J.D.A.: Further studies in the therapeutic value of lysergic acid diethylamide in mental illness. *J Ment Sci, 103*:332, 1957.
5. ABRAMSON, H.A.; JARVIK, M.E.; KAUFMAN, M.R.; KORNETSKY, C.; LEVINE, A., and WAGNER, M.: Lysergic acid diethylamide (LSD 25). I: Physiological and perceptual responses. *J Psychol, 39*:3, 1955.
6. ABRAMSON, H. A.: Lysergic acid diethylamide (LSD 25). XXIX: The response index as a measure of threshold activity of psychotropic drugs in man. *J Psychol, 48*:65, 1959.
7. ABRAMSON, H.A.: Lysergic acid diethylamide (LSD 25). XXXI: Comparison by questionnaire of psychotomimetic activities of congeners on normal subjects and drug addicts. *J Ment Sci, 106*:1120, 1960.
8. ABRAMSON, H.A.; JARVIK, M.E.; LEVINE, A.; KAUFMAN, M.R., and HIRSCH, M.W.: Lysergic acid diethylamide (LSD 25). The effects produced by substitution of a tap water placebo. *J Psychol, 40*:367, 1955.
9. ABRAMSON, H.A., *et al.*: Lysergic acid diethylamide (LSD 25). XVII: Tolerance development and its relationship to the theory of psychosis. *J Psychol, 41*:81, 1956.
10. ABRAMSON, H.A. (Ed.): *The Use of LSD in Psychotherapy.* New York, Josiah Macy Jr. Foundation, 1960.
11. ABRAMSON, H.A. (Ed.): *The Use of LSD in Psychotherapy and Alcoholism.* Indianapolis, Bobbs, 1967.
12. FREDERKING, W.: Intoxicant drugs (LSD-25) and mescaline in psychotherapy. *J Nerv Ment Dis, 121*:262-266, 1955.
13. SAVAGE, C.; HARMAN, W.W.; FADIMAN, J., and SAVAGE, E.: An evaluation of the psychedelic experience. Presented at Annual Meeting, American Psychiatric Association, St. Louis, May 9, 1963.
14. SAVAGE, C.; TERRILL, J., and JACKSON, D.D.: LSD transcendence and the new beginning. *J Nerv Ment Dis, 135*:425, 1962.
15. BENDER, L.; FARETRA, G., and COBRINK, L.: LSD and UML treatment of hospitalized disturbed children. *Recent Advances Biol Psychia, 5*:84, 1963.

16. SIMMONS, J.Q.; LEIKEN, S.J.; LOVAAS, O.I.; SCHAEFFER, B., and PERLOFF, B.: Modification of autistic behavior with LSD-25. *Amer J Psychiat.*

17. VAN DUSEN, W.; WILSON, W.; MINERS, W., and HOOK, H.: Treatment of alcoholism with lysergide. *Quart J Stud Alcohol, 28:*295-304, 1967.

18. O'REILLY, P., and REICH, G.: Lysergic acid and the alcoholic. *Dis Nerv Syst, 23:*331-334, 1962.

19. SMITH, C.M.: A new adjunct to the treatment of alcoholism: The hallucinogenic drugs. *Quart J Stud Alcohol, 19:*406, 1958.

20. CHWELOS, N.; BLEWETT, D.B., SMITH, C.M., and HOFFER, A.: Use of d-lysergic acid diethylamide in the treatment of alcoholism. *Quart J Stud Alcohol, 20:*577-590, 1959.

21. DITMAN, K.S.; HAYMAN, M., and WHITTLESEY, J.R.B.: Nature and frequency of claims following LSD. *J Nerv Ment Dis, 134:*4, 1962.

22. DITMAN, K., and BAILEY, J.J.: Evaluating LSD as a psychotherapeutic agent. In *The Use of LSD in Psychotherapy and and Alcoholism.* Indianapolis, Bobbs, 1967, vol. III, p. 154.

23. GROF, S.: Use of LSD 25 in personality diagnostics and therapy of psychogenic disorders. In *The Use of LSD in Psychotherapy and Alcoholism.* Indianapolis, Bobbs, 1967, vol. III, p. 154.

24. WOLPE, J.: *Psychotherapy by Reciprocal Inhibition.* Stanford, Stanford, 1958.

25. MARTIN, A.: LSD (lysergic acid diethylamide) treatment of chronic psychoneurotic patients under day-hospital conditions. *Int J. Soc Psychiat, 3:*188, 1957.

26. BUCKMAN, J.: Theoretical aspects of LSD therapy. In *The Use of LSD in Psychotherapy and Alcoholism.* Indianapolis, Bobbs, 1967, vol. III, p. 83.

27. VAN RHIJN, C.H.: Symbolysis: Psychotherapy by symbolic presentation. In ABRAMSON, H.A. (Ed.) : *The Use of LSD in Psychotherapy.* New York, Josiah Macy, Jr. Foundation, 1960.

28. VAN RHIJN, C.H.: Variables in psycholytic treatment. In *The Use of LSD in Psychotherapy and Alcoholism.* Indianapolis, Bobbs, 1967, vol. III, p. 208.

29. NEWLAND, C.: *Myself and I.* New York, Coward McCann, 1962.

30. MOSS, T.: Personal Communication.

31. LEUNER, H.: Present state of psycholytic thearpy and its possibilities. *The Use of LSD in Psychotherapy and Alcoholism.* Indianapolis, Bobbs, 1967, vol. III, p. 101.

32. GROF, S.: Tentative theoretical framework for understanding dynamics of LSD psychotherapy. Private circulation, 1966.

33. MOGAR, R.E., and SAVAGE, C.: Personality change associated with psychedelic (LSD) therapy. *Psychotherapy, 1:*64-73, 1964.

34. COHEN, S., and DITMAN, K.S.: Complications associated with lysergic acid diethylamide (LSD-25). *JAMA, 181:*161-162, 1962.

35. UNGERLEIDER, J.T.; FISHER, D.D., and FULLER, M.: The dangers of LSD. *JAMA, 197:*389-392, 1966.

36. GRINKER, R.R.: Bootlegged ecstasy. *JAMA, 187:*768, 1964.

37. LING, T.M., and BUCKMAN, J.: *Lysergic acid (LSD 25) and Ritalin in the treatment of neurosis.* Sidcup, Kent, England, Lombardo Press, 1963.

38. DITMAN, K.S., *et al.: Experimental Effects of LSD-25, Methylphenidate and Chlordiazepoxide with Alcoholics* (in press) 1967.

39. DITMAN, K.S., *et al.: Harmful Aspects of the LSD Experience,* 1967 (in press).

40. COHEN, M.M.; MARINELLO, M.J., and BACK, N.: *Science, 155:*1417, 1967.

41. IRWIN, S., *et al.:* Presented at the American Psychiatric Association, Annual Meeting, 1967.

42. ALEXANDER, G.J., *et al.:* LSD: Injection early in pregnancy produces abnormalities in offspring of rats. *Science, 157:*3787, 1967.

Chapter IV

THE ACUTE SIDE EFFECTS FROM LSD

J. THOMAS UNGERLEIDER

INTRODUCTION

There are a number of physiologic effects often seen following LSD ingestion which one would not call side effects. These effects include both a reported loss of appetite and an increased appetite, dilated pupils, transient chilliness, flushing of the skin, and transient increases in blood pressure, pulse rate and blood sugar. The most common symptoms in patients presenting at UCLA's Neuropsychiatric Institute following LSD ingestion have been (in decreasing order of frequency) frightening auditory and visual hallucinations, anxiety to the point of panic, depression (often with suicidal thoughts and some suicide attempts, some severe) and confusion—people wandering about, not knowing where they were (1). Paranoid reactions are also common, and even seizures have been reported (2).

It is important to emphasize however that the above symptoms are frequently experienced as a part of or a reaction to the perceptual changes which regularly follow the ingestion of LSD. For the term *psychedelic,* meaning mind-manifesting, refers to the intensification of sensation and distortion of perception under LSD. Thus, whether the acute effects from LSD are called a "freak trip," "bummer" or "freak out," as LSD users describe a bad LSD experience, has not only to do with the perceptual alteration itself but with the user's reaction to it.

Many persons have experienced some or all of the above effects (hallucinations, anxiety, depression, confusion and paranoia) after taking LSD but claimed to be able to get over them either by themselves or with the use of a "sitter" or guide. Thus they never sought aid and were not thought of as suffering from the acute side effects of the drug. However, other users have reacted strongly and adversely to experiencing these perceptual changes under LSD and have sought psychiatric or medical aid either directly or indirectly. (Many of the chronic LSD users who have been leading nomadic lives manage, when they begin to have a bad trip, to find their way home to their parents whom they know perfectly well will seek medical aid for them. Nonetheless, these patients usually present at a medical or psychiatric facility claiming that they are not suffering and that they are only there because their parents brought them.)

Under LSD each person has a highly personalized experience. Some people say they can "hear colors" and others "see sounds." Some people experience mystical or semi-religious feelings under LSD. Illusory phenomena are common. For example, one man slept on the floor the night he took LSD because he was convinced his bed was only two inches long. Another man was restrained from diving off a cliff onto the rocks in the ocean below. Later he explained that he thought the breaking waves were a silk scarf and he wanted to dive into it and roll on it. Faces may appear to be melting. One high school student cut all the flexor tendons in her wrist when she looked in the mirror and saw her face begin to dissolve. Time sense is especially distorted. We have seen persons under the influence of LSD stare at their fingers or at a leaf for hours (3) .

Delusions are not infrequent. We treated, in crisis intervention, a young man who became convinced, a few hours after ingesting LSD for the first time, that he had to offer a human sacrifice, that is kill someone or die himself. He was prevented from throwing his girlfriend off the roof of a

Hollywood hotel. Another user developed a delusional system about colors. He believed that green vapors were coming from the air into his umbilicus and that everything red in his house was harmful to him. He threw away every red item at home, including food and furniture.

THE TRIP ITSELF

There are some common features which occur at LSD "happenings," whether it is two or sixty users taking the drug together. There is usually a period of anywhere from one to three hours after the drug begins to take effect (one-half hour to forty-five minutes after ingestion) where the user lies perfectly still as though asleep. He may, however, also be sitting or occasionally reading. Following this period of time, many users become more active and begin to walk and particularly to seek outdoor surroundings. They may stare at their finger or at a leaf or a shadow for hours on end. They frequently talk to themselves, laugh or giggle, and are quite passive and suggestible. They may say "Do you see it? Isn't it beautiful?" over and over, to which the other users often will chant in unison, "Yes we see it."

The effects usually wear off in twelve to sixteen hours, but occasionally they may persist for days or even weeks. Most users take LSD only once or twice a week because of the rapid development of tolerance. The onset of effects is independent of the route of administration so persons rarely take LSD intravenously unless emotionally addicted to needles. Sexual experiences while on a trip are extremely rare. As one person put it so well, "Why waste something as good as LSD on something as common as sex" (4, 5).

There is no lethal overdosage from LSD reported in humans. The main direct fatality so far was an elephant who died from an overdose when he was given 0.15 *milligrams* of LSD per kilogram of body weight (297 mg) in an experimental situation.

PREDICTABILITY

The occurrence of acute side effects from LSD *cannot* be predicted. Psychiatric interviews and psychological testing do *not* screen out adverse reactors. Some of the worst reactions have been in persons, often physicians and other professionals, who appeared stable by every indicator. Conversely, others who have had histories of severe psychiatric problems and have been leading marginal existences have seemed to tolerate massive daily doses of LSD without ill effect. There is some work to show that persons who place a premium on self-control, planning, caution and impulse restriction and who sacrifice spontaneity do particularly poorly on LSD.

Many persons have their freak trip the first time they take the drug. Others have as many as 150 previous good experiences first. It is important to note that *recurrence* of the acute side effects from LSD in all their original intensity often appears up to eighteen months after ingestion of the drug, either with stress or without apparent stress, *without* further ingestion of any LSD.

DIFFERENTIAL DIAGNOSIS

It is important to rule out the paranoid schizophrenic (they are beginning to present in emergency rooms complaining of having been poisoned by LSD by their persecutors). Upon investigation they usually have chronic histories of mental illness. In addition, they know little about LSD and have not been to any of the few places where it might be placed in their drink without their knowledge (i.e., an "acid test" partly). Most LSD users realize the danger of giving the drug to an unprepared person, and thus the likelihood of this happening is minimal.

It is difficult to keep abreast of the many new substances which keep appearing and are alleged to have psychedelic properties. The most recent, and potentially most significant, is a heterogenous group of compounds loosely called STP (not to be confused with the oil additive). One of the compounds called STP is apparently a mixture of several psychedelics, including LSD, DMT (dimethyl tryptamine), psilocybin and peyote. Another substance, also called STP, has been identified as an atropinelike drug originally developed by the Army as a chemical warfare agent. It has been variously known as JB 314, BZ and Ditran.

This is not the first time that atropine derivatives have appeared on the black market and have been ingested for their hallucinatory effects (1). Atropine poisoning long has been known to produce dry mouth, dilated pupils, blurred vision, tachycardia and temperature elevation (skin dry and flushed). There may be difficulty swallowing as well as disturbances of gait and speech. Mental alterations include disturbance in memory, disorientation, hallucinations (especially visual), mania and delirium. Death may occur due to respiratory failure. The full-blown picture of atropine poisoning is thus not difficult to distinguish from LSD's side effects which are essentially restricted to the mental manifestations previously described. Although with LSD the sensorium is usually clear and illusions (rather than true hallucinations) are the rule, delirious and hallucinatory states are now being reported with increasing frequency.

It is important that a person suffering from atropine poisoning not be treated with chlorpromazine (the drug of choice for an LSD reaction) because the peripheral cholinergic blocking activity of chlorpromazine potentiates the atropine effects.

Intravenous physostigmine has been theoretically suggested to counteract the atropinelike activity of STP, although no reports of its clinical effectiveness have yet been reported.

TREATMENT

Treatment of the acute symptoms first must be directed towards preventing the patient from physically harming himself or others. Thus the frequent indication for psychiatric hospitalization. We use interpersonal rather than mechanical restraints. Warm support and reassurance are usually quite effective. The patient should be encouraged to relax and *not* try to differentiate which perceptions are real and which are due to the drug's effect. As the guides say, "flow with it."

Chemical agents are also a vital part of the treatment regime. Chlorpromazine (Thorazine) is the most effective antagonist to LSD effects, both clinically and experimentally (6). A 50 mg test dose of Thorazine followed by 100 to 150 mg every four to six hours orally or parenterally for several days is usually effective. The effectiveness is seen clinically by a reversal of the hallucinations and other side effects and can also be demonstrated by reversibility of the electroencephalographic changes (7). This antagonistic effect of chlorpromazine can also be demonstrated in animal experiments (8). In contrast, reserpine may actually enhance the effects of LSD. Barbiturates may have some antagonistic effect on LSD as may azacyclonal (Frenquel®).

It should be emphasized however that chlorpromazine is not always effective in treating of LSD complications.

> CASE REPORT: A twenty-two-year-old single white man became psychotic approximately twenty-four hours after the ingestion of LSD. He had both auditory and visual hallucinations. He had use LSD once before without difficulty. Several parenteral doses of 50 mg chlorpromazine plus orally administered chlorpromazine up to 2000 mg per day and chlorpromazine in conjunction with trifluoperazine hydrochloride (Stelazine®) resulted in no reduction or improvement of the psychosis. The patient improved slowly after a period of six weeks. Improvement was seemingly unrelated to the phenothiazine medication.

PSYCHOTHERAPY

Psychotherapy in the acute stage of LSD intoxication consists particularly of reassurance. This is what the LSD guide or sitter does. It is directed at convincing the patient that he has not permanently harmed himself and that the effects will wear off. He should never be told that he has "irreparably damaged his brain" (as one LSD user was told when he called an emergency facility for crisis intervention. This promptly precipitated a panic). The patient should not try to fight to regain his perceptual discrimination by attempting to distinguish what is real and what is not real at the moment. Rather, he should try to relax. Because the LSD user is quite suggestible this approach is usually extremely effective.

It is important also not to physically intrude upon the calm LSD user while he is under the influence of the drug. He is usually very passive unless in a panic, and will rarely harm anyone even when provoked. Violence and homicide are most rare. Police who try to handcuff and arrest someone who is "on a trip" do sometimes manage to provoke violence however. Conversely, one cannot permit a panicky patient to remain out of control and be destructive. If talking and reassurance are not effective, physical restraint may eventually be required.

Psychotherapy on a long-term basis should be directed to finding out why the particular person prefers a drugged solution to life's problems. Particular conflict areas frequently have to do with rebelliousness and inability to tolerate the feelings of sexuality and aggression as well as inability to handle the daily frustrations and anxieties of living.

PROGNOSIS

Although most persons respond promptly to intervention from their acute adverse LSD reaction, many users do return to these drugs. They seem naive and assume that they either will not have another bad experience or that if they mix LSD with some other drug, particularly marijuana and/or one of the new memory drugs or other psychedelics, they will then be able to find the proper combination which will insure a happy frustration-free life.

Bibliography

1. UNGERLEIDER, J. T.; FISHER, D., and FULLER, M.: The dangers of LSD. *JAMA, 197*:109-112, 1966.
2. FISHER, D., and UNGERLEIDER, J. T.: Grand mal seizures after LSD ingestion. *Calif Med, 106*:210-211, 1967.
3. UNGERLEIDER, J. T., and FISHER, D.: The problems of LSD-25 and emotional disorder. *Calif Med, 106*:49-55, 1967.
4. UNGERLEIDER, J. T., and FISHER, D.: LSD: Research and joyride. *The Nation,* May 16, 1966.
5. UNGERLEIDER, J. T., and FISHER, D.: LSD: Fact and fantasy, *Arts and Architecture, 83*:18-20, 1966.
6. CLARK, L. D., and BLISS, E. L.: Psychopharmacological studies of lysergic acid diethylamide (LSD) intoxication. *Arch Neurol Psychiat, 78*:653-655, 1957.
7. MONROE, R. R.; HEATH, R. C.; MICKLE, W. A., and LLEWELLYN, R.C.: Correlation of rhinencephalic electrograms with behavior: A study on humans under the influence of LSD and mescaline. *Electro enceph Clin Neurophysiol,* 9:623-642, 1957.
8. STURTEVANT, F. M., and DRILL, V. A.: Effects of mescaline in laboratory animals and influence of ataraxics on mescaline response. *Proc Soc Exp Biol Med, 92*:383-387, 1956.

Chapter V

THE CHRONIC SIDE EFFECTS FROM LSD

DUKE D. FISHER

The previous chapter has dealt with some of the acute side effects that occur after taking LSD. For the past several years there has been a growing focus among newspapers, magazines and other news media on some of the more bizarre, acute effects from LSD. In addition there has been increasing attention to some of the long-term effects of LSD usage. These effects include changes in personality, motivation and attitudes. These chronic side effects from LSD have been noticed by many psychiatrists, psychiatric residents, and other medical practitioners as well as clinical psychologists, social workers, and others who have been seeing patients who have used LSD in various dosages and frequency and have developed certain long-term changes. This chapter will deal with the more frequently observed chronic untoward reactions to LSD.

RECURRENCE OF LSD EXPERIENCE

One of the most frequently reported chronic side effects from LSD is the recurrence of a portion of the original LSD experience without using the drug again (1,2). We have seen many patients at UCLA who have used LSD in a wide dosage range and varying frequency and have recurrences of portions of the LSD experience as much as eighteen months later without using the drug again. Many times the recurrence is described as occurring in the original intensity, but the length of time seems to be much less, varying from a few seconds to two or three hours. Most of the recurrences seem to diminish in intensity and frequency with the passage of time. Many of the recurrences have to do with paranoid thoughts, hallucinatory activity, and feelings of unreality and estrangement that were experienced during the original LSD induced episode.

> CASE REPORT: A twenty-two-year-old white male was admitted to UCLA as an inpatient, primarily because of recurrences of LSD-induced paranoid ideation. He had used LSD on one occasion and experienced the feeling that someone was going to kill him. The remainder of the LSD experience was quite typical of those described by LSD users. Two months after the original LSD experience, the patient was on a date with his girlfriend and, during an argument, suddenly had what he described as a "flashback" in which he suddenly had the thought that his girlfriend was going to kill him. He become frightened, and after this experience occurred several more times, decided to seek psychiatric help. In addition to the paranoid ideation, the patient also experienced observing the melting of faces and a feeling of oneness that had also occurred when he initially took the LSD. The patient had no previous psychiatric history and denied any paranoid ideation or drug use prior to using the LSD.

In this case, the recurrence of the LSD experience seemed to be precipitated by stress, namely certain times in which there would be an argument between the patient and his girlfriend. However, we have seen cases in which there seemed to be no apparent stress. These cases have included the transient appearance of walls pulsating, faces melting, or panic states while walking to work, driving on the freeway, or resting at home. One young lady had a particularly distressing problem while driving on the freeway in the evening. She would experience flashbacks and a pair of headlights from an oncoming car would seem so bright and intense as to become a hundred headlights. She would then experience a feeling of panic as she tried to distinguish which were the two *real* headlights.

Some LSD users maintain they can precipitate the LSD recurrence by using marijuana. It should also be noted that some LSD users maintain that they can precipitate pleasurable or desirable LSD-like experiences merely by listening to certain forms of music, or from other nondrug stimuli.

VALUE SYSTEM CHANGES

Certainly we are aware that many chronic drug users are not considered the most ardent enthusiasts or promotors of what are considered socially productive endeavors. Some individuals who use LSD describe a dramatic shift in their value system (3). This usually has to do with being much less interested in work and having more interest in and preoccupation with LSD, mysticism or other experimental components of the LSD trip. Some of the users of LSD explain that they develop an insight that enables them to see through the "ego games" of society. "Turn on, tune in, and drop out"—the phrase popularized by Dr. Timothy Leary seems to be an accurate description of an observable phenomenon after many people use LSD. Many users of LSD, who have returned to work, admitted an inability to concentrate, lack of motivation, and a preoccupation with fantasy that made it virtually impossible for them to work. Some of these individuals indicated that during this period of time they rationalized their difficulty working by claiming a new kind of insight.

Since some of the young people who use LSD had previously been involved in various active movements including antiwar activity, social protest, etc., it has been interesting to note that many of them, after using LSD, still pay lip service to some of their goals. However, they become much less active in terms of doing anything toward achieving social or political reforms. We interviewed a gentleman who since taking LSD found himself much less interested in his law studies and more interested in ruminating alone in his room for hours about the possibility of forming an organization that would "turn on" LBJ or Mao Tse Tung so that we might have world peace.

We have spoken to many high school and college students who have dropped out of school after using LSD, maintaining that "school is no longer challenging." There have also been professional people, business men, artists and lawyers who have decided that their former pursuits are now without meaning after taking LSD.

SUBJECTIVE FEELING OF IMPROVEMENT WITH OBJECTIVE LOSS OF FUNCTIONING

Many of the patients brought for treatment to UCLA were accompanied by families, friends, or interested parties who seemed much more concerned about the effects than did the LSD patient. In fact, many of the LSD patients maintained that "things were never better." Some LSD users even claimed new kinds of power such as extrasensory perception, the ability to pick up vibrations from people and read minds, improvement in school without studying, and new problem-solving abilities. We evaluated some of these claims of improvement and new powers and found that there occurs on a chronic basis among many users of LSD a *subjective* feeling of improvement but an *objective* loss of functioning (3). We saw one young drummer who felt he was playing as well as Gene Krupa; however, his business manager who brought him to our facility maintained that he was in danger of losing his job since none of the other band members could accompany him and no one could dance to his music. We did some longitudinal studies on several students who maintained that they had improved their abilities to learn after using LSD; however, we found that they had either dropped out of school or dropped some of their courses, many times with lower grade averages. When we questioned the students they informed us that their learning powers were so intense that school no longer had meaning for them. This feeling of omnipotence concerning one's abilities included one gentleman who claimed great problem-solving ability but who had lost his job as a mathematical engineer because of his inability to do effective calculations. We worked with one young group which maintained "ESP awareness" after using LSD. Some members of the group offered to demonstrate their ESP powers by reading the minds of other group members only to find that they could do no better than they would have by chance alone.

This feeling of omnipotence and resultant unwarranted self-confidence has been described with other hallucinogenic drugs, including marijuana (4). As mentioned initially, this type of euphoria and feeling of omnipotence has resulted in many LSD users seeking treatment only at the insistence of friends, families, or by court order. It is rather apparent after talking with many LSD users that beneath this feeling of omnipotence is a great feeling of helplessness and fear of loss of control. Some of the LSD users who have remained in treatment have admitted to being frightened of being overwhelmed by the LSD experience or by their surroundings. Some of the LSD mythology (which includes the false notions that doubling the dose will terminate a bad trip, or that taking LSD while holding certain kinds of religious symbols will prevent a complication) is an attempt to handle the loss of control and feelings of helplessness that occur after using this very powerful drug. Unfortunately, unless this feeling of omnipotence is rapidly dealt with in therapy, it is most difficult to keep the LSD patient in treatment.

INTERPERSONAL RELATIONSHIPS

One of the chronic side effects from using LSD seems to occur in the area of interpersonal relationships. Many LSD patients attend "love-ins," "love sessions," and other events emphasizing and including the word *love*. Many chronic LSD users talk about love a great deal. Many of the symbols of the LSD subculture have to do with flowers, bells and peace symbols. Interestingly enough, however, the love seems to be a highly narcissistic, objectless love. Most of the LSD users have a great deal of difficulty loving *one* other person. They seem to have difficulty tolerating the feelings that occur with closeness. Freud's description of primary narcissism, in which he describes this noncathecting type of self-love, is particularly applicable to the LSD user (5). One generally witnesses an increasing difficulty with interpersonal relationships among users of LSD. They attempt to play the "game of love" without meeting the demands, risks, and vicissitudes of a close relationship with another person. Some of the love sessions that we attended were impressive in terms of the number of monologues taking place. Many of the LSD users are not concerned about the other members of the group as much as they are preoccupied with the intensity of their own internal experiences. It seems that the devotion to the word love that is found among many groups who use LSD is really a counterphobic attempt to deal with the very closeness that many of them cannot tolerate.

USE OF LSD BY THE ADOLESCENT

There is no question that a great deal of LSD usage is among adolescents. Much of the initial appeal to adolescents seems to be that LSD lends itself so well to their identity struggles. Since most adolescents are quite concerned about who they are, where they are going, and what is really important in life, they are quite curious concerning the claims made by proselytizers of LSD. These claims include the allegation that LSD provides instant insight, instant knowledge, and instant ability to see the world as it really is.

In addition to this appeal, many of the adolescents who use

LSD on a chronic basis do so in an attempt to avoid their feelings of aggression and sexuality. Many of the adolescents who continue LSD usage are those who have particular difficulty accommodating their feelings of aggression and sexuality. Most people, while on LSD, are quite passive, suggestible, and rarely concerned about sex or anger. Some of them who laud the LSD effects maintain that they don't have to get "hung up" with sexual matters or hostile feelings. Unfortunately, it is at this very time of life that the adolescent is faced with the task of finding ways to master and deal with his feelings of sexuality and aggression; consequently, the chronic use of LSD enables one to create the psychedelic or drugged effect in lieu of experiencing one's own instinctual feelings. In a sense, the chronic use of LSD among the adolescent robs him of a chance to grow up emotionally.

MISSIONARY QUALITY

Many LSD users do not merely take the drug themselves but insist that their families, their friends, and anyone close to them use LSD. This is not an uncommon phenomenon among drug users in general; however, I have been especially impressed by the missionary quality that seems to persist with the LSD user. What is especially alarming, however, is that some professionals, who have done work with LSD and have used it themselves, seem to find it increasingly difficult to be objective about the drug and tend to glamorize LSD while refusing to consider some of the adverse side effects of the drug. This missionary aspect in LSD users has become an increasing problem with young mothers who insist on giving LSD to their children. Some mothers who have been "turning on" their children are now beginning to express concern since publication of the recent study that indicates increases in chromosomal aberration in human leukocytes of individuals who have taken LSD (6).

PERSISTENT PSYCHOSIS

A consideration of the chronic effects of LSD should include the prolonged psychosis. This persistent psychotic pattern has been described in the literature (3,7). The prolonged psychotic reaction usually includes fragmentary ego-functioning with inappropriate affect, hallucinations and loosening of associations. Many times the picture is very much like that of schizophrenia. However, other patients present with the confusion, vivid visual hallucinatory activity, and disorientation more characteristic of a toxic psychosis. We have seen instances of borderline psychotics who have become grossly schizophrenic after using LSD. Some patients have had to be transferred to state hospitals because of the prolonged psychosis; others have cleared with the use of phenothiazines, long-term hospitalization and, in some instances, electroshock treatment. The use of chlorpromazine in the treatment of the acute LSD psychosis has been previously described in Chapter IV of this book.

DIFFERENTIAL DIAGNOSIS

In dealing with some of the chronic effects of LSD it is important to carefully assess the premorbid personality of the LSD user and the concomitant use of other drugs. Some of the aforementioned chronic effects are observed to some degree in the personality types that tend to use a variety of drugs, including the amphetamines, barbiturates and narcotics. However, we have found that LSD is unique in that some people develop the personality changes on a single dose of LSD. Individuals with well-integrated personalities and no previous psychiatric histories have also developed some of the chronic effects after LSD usage.

Another factor that must be considered is that many LSD users identify themselves with certain hippie subcultures in which withdrawal from society and a nonaggressive approach toward life are held in high esteem. Since many LSD users are quite suggestible after using the drug, they rapidly adopt the social values of various subcultures in which drug usage is quite prevalent. It is also important to obtain a detailed history of drug use. We have seen members of the hippie subculture who describe psychedelic experience such as perceptual changes and frank hallucinations *without* using drugs. There are other reported instances of psychedelic experiences in groups where drugs are not used (8). The parallels between the LSD subject and the good hypnotic subject are striking, particularly in the realm of passivity and suggestibility.

TREATMENT

Treatment considerations include a careful assessment of the state of ego functioning. Many of the patients displaying chronic LSD effects are functioning with a psychotic or borderline psychotic ego state. On the other hand, many neurotics and character disorders display certain of the chronic effects mentioned.

The previously mentioned recurrence phenomenon can sometimes be quite refractory in terms of treatment. I have found personally that the use of Stelaziner® or Mellaril® coupled with psychotherapy can be quite helpful. Some patients seem to respond to treatment with a diminished frequency and intensity of LSD recurrences. Many times a person's subjective reaction to the recurrences is extremely important and reassurance by the therapist that the recurrences will diminish in time in terms of frequency and intensity can be quite reassuring.

Some patients who have special difficulty at work, on freeways, or other places where the recurrence can be a social problem must be warned and directed by the therapist to either avoid these circumstances or make arrangements to accommodate them. Some patients have fears that the recurrences will persist forever or that they are becoming permanently psychotic. I know of no reported cases of the *recurrence* leading to a prolonged psychosis; hence I feel that the therapist can safely reassure the patient that this does not seem to be a permanent personality change.

Unfortunately many times the dramatic changes in value systems and subjective feelings of improvement with an objective loss of functioning results in LSD patients being brought to treatment by an interested party or family member. In this case the task of therapy is to interest the patient in becoming involved in psychotherapy himself. The relationship with the therapist seems to be crucial. Some of the LSD users that we have spoken with had a great deal of contempt and little confidence in therapists who identified with LSD users and considered themselves "hippie therapists." On the other hand, a very strict authoritarian approach is quickly dismissed as being offered by a "tool of the establishment." Since many patients who have used LSD have great difficulty in tolerating their own feelings and prefer the drugged state from LSD, it is important to convey to them the acceptability of their hostile feelings as well as their warm and tender feelings. Many times it is useful to approach the use of LSD as a defense against life and attempt to determine what it is about their existence that is so unpleasant that the use of LSD is necessary. The nature of treatment varies considerably since LSD users range from the curious neurotic to the severely disturbed schizophrenic patient.

PROGNOSIS

My experience has been that many of the patients who remain in treatment do quite well, providing they don't continue to use LSD. Unfortunately, many LSD users displaying the aforementioned chronic effects of the drug leave treatment and continue to use LSD in an attempt to find a magic solution to their problems. There is a great deal of magical thinking that goes into the use of LSD, and the many users of LSD who cannot tolerate difficulties of a search within themselves prefer to attempt magical solutions by the continued use of LSD. The many patients who are forced into treatment by parents, families, the authorities or friends are usually not motivated for any kind of treatment, and unless a motivation is developed for some type of help the prognosis is very guarded.

Bibliography

1. UNGERLEIDER, J.T., and FISHER, D.: LSD: Research and joyride. *The Nation,* May 16, 1966.
2. COOPER, H.A.: Hallucinogenic drugs. *Lancet, 268*:1078, 1955.
3. UNGERLEIDER, J.T., and FISHER, D.: The problems of LSD[25] and emotional disorder. *Calif Med, 106*:49-55, 1967.
4. BLOOMQUIST, E.R.: Marijuana: Social benefit or social detriment? *Calif Med, 106*:346-353.
5. FREUD, S.: *Collected Papers.* London, Hogarth, 1948, vol. 4, pp. 30-60.
6. COHEN, M.M., and MARINELLO, M.J.: Chromosomal damage in human leukocytes induced by lysergic acid diethylamide. *Science, 155*:1417, 1967.
7. COHEN, S.: Lysergic acid diethylamide: Side effects and complications. *J Nerv Ment Dis, 130*:35-36, 1960.
8. The psychedelic game. *Mademoiselle,* March, 1966, p. 179.

Chapter VI

THE PROSPECTS OF LSD

Opinion of J. Thomas Ungerleider

The prospects for legitimate use of LSD are dismal as of this date. The LSD hysteria continues to increase and it is not confined to the general public and mass media alone. Professionals are just as unscientific. Examples of hysteria among the press and public are legion.

One Los Angeles paper recently features headlines about confiscation of a huge lot of LSD. The retraction, several weeks later and buried in the back of the paper, stated merely that the substance turned out to be sugar.

Two of the contributors to this volume reported *one case* of LSD induced grand mal seizures in a brief communication in the state medical journal. It made headlines in the San Francisco newspapers and was picked up by a national news service. LSD was trumpeted throughout the country as a cause of epilepsy.

Recently there was a tragedy in a mental hospital where two of the contributors work (a tragedy having nothing to do with drugs or the authors). The news media immediately called to ask if they could feature the incident as an "LSD murder."

The press also falls prey to becoming threatened, then defensive, and finally retaliatory against this apparently inexplicable behavior of the adolescent.

Our younger generation's drugged search for El Dorado

and nirvana in a capsule is increasing. Last month featured "mellow-yellow" (banana skins) and "DMT" (dimethyltryptamine). This week alone I have received half a dozen calls (including several from the East Coast) from the press about STP, an as yet chemically unidentified psychedelic. An article has just arrived in our state medical journal about nitrous oxide inhalation for kicks, and the radio today featured wheat as the latest "turn on." Everyone is concerned, as parents look for help, but no one knows what to do. Many educators are wrestling with the problem. The superintendent of schools of our state recently stated that LSD is the most pressing problem in our high schools today.

Two of us (D.D.F. and J.T.U.) have been spending a great deal of time speaking about LSD to youngsters in schools, colleges and church groups (approximately 200 lectures to over 100,000 college and high school students throughout California over the past 2 years.) Although our emphasis is on LSD, many youngsters ask questions about the effects of marijuana. Because we have not ourselves seen persons in trouble from marijuana, either at our hospital or in our community "explorations," we cannot speak first-hand about its effects. But unfortunately we often find that these youngsters have been told, particularly by narcotics officers, that since marijuana and LSD are both hallucinogens, they are thus both equally deadly. Yet most scientific investigators agree that LSD is hundreds to thousands of times more harmful than marijuana.

And because marijuana offenses are felonies and LSD possession is a misdemeanor, they may have been told that "pot" is worse than "acid." This is unfortunate because these youngsters, seeing through such obvious distortions, then not only reject all of these things adults have said about marijuana but they *also reject* what is said about LSD's dangers. This is a real tragedy.

The police, narcotic officers and government officials are

just as perplexed. The LSD antipossession laws are hard, if not impossible, to enforce. Thus a wide variety of opinions are held. I have been particularly impressed by the usually sensitive and thoughtful position and behavior of law enforcement in the Los Angeles area, on city, state and Federal levels.

Yet wide discrepancies do exist. At a drug abuse panel on which I participated in a large California city this spring, the local police chief announced to the audience that he was out to "get" *not only* the drug abusers and lawbreakers but also "those kids with long hair and funny shoes." At a mayor's youth council meeting recently, a city attorney advised the youths that the real problem was the way today's youngsters *experimented with new ideas.* (This he added could *even* lead to reading of pornography!)

Dr. Fisher and I had a chance to observe the police frustration firsthand when, enroute to and in the environs of a love-in, our car was stopped by a police officer. We were informally attired, and obviously mistaking us for love-in participants and not "scientific observers," the officer was extremely rude, shouted at us and behaved in a manner which was unlike any we (as solid citizens) had ever witnessed. When we identified ourselves the officer's manner changed immediately and he stated, "I'm only an honest cop trying to do my job." We had already been ticketed, but subsequently asked for an investigation, and the charges were dropped because of certain "irregularities" in the issuance of the citation.

The lack of objectivity is no better among the professional and medical communities. I have just refused an invitation to appear on a *physician*—professional drug abuse panel in Los Angeles which is advertised as featuring a film that "exposes the supposedly innocent 'love-ins' and true 'happenings' for what they are—traps of filth and perversion for our youth." The brochure connects increased drug abuse in Southern California with the playing of the songs "Rainy

Day Woman," "Eight Miles High," "Tomorrow Never Knows," "Crystal Ships" and "Acapulco Gold" on United States radio stations. It implicates the smoking of banana skins (although acknowledging that they have *no* drug effect) as leading to the use of LSD and marijuana. Lenin and Marx are, of course, implicated.

Before a recent panel on LSD, two of us heard the co-investigator of a large study on LSD use (soon to begin via Federal grant) admit that both he and the principal investigator had been LSD users. The researcher was then told by the regional head of another Federal agency that *every result* he would publish would now be discounted by the agency because he was an LSD user and therefore no longer able to be objective. And The New York Medical Society recently declared LSD to be more deadly than *heroin.*

On the other hand, both Dr. Fisher and I have been told, both in public and in private and by professionals and physicians (and seriously) that we do not understand the *true dignity* of the San Francisco (Haight-Ashbury) hippies. Their drug use, we are told, is no real problem but represents an eloquent protest to Vietnam, and for civil rights and the like. This is in marked contrast to all other hippies, particularly to the hippies at the very bottom of the pecking order, the Los Angeles (i.e. Hollywood) hippies. (Thus the traditional Los Angeles-San Francisco rivalry has even been applied to the LSD problem.)

Or, on a recent panel before a widely cheering pro-LSD crowd, one of our contributors abandoned his usual objectivity and stated, "Anyone who can hold his alcohol can hold his LSD"—more applause.

Last week I watched a television interview of a young physician who works in the Haight-Ashbury district of San Francisco. It was part of a popular teen-age show, *Groovy,* filmed on the beach in Los Angeles and was brought to my attention by the neighborhood children. The physician was asked if there was any truth to the chromosome damage reports from LSD. His entire answer was that the problem was "due to the adults' fear about LSD because it makes you more artistic and adults want you to work from '8 to 5' on dull and boring jobs."

This heated controversy ranges even inside the psychiatric profession. At the recent National Convention of the American Psychiatric Association in Detroit, Michigan, the controversy reached new highs. Two confirmatory and as yet unpublished studies of the chromosomal alterations in white blood cells of LSD users were inserted into the program (one from Portland, Oregon and one from Bellevue Hospital in New York). This set the tenor for the LSD part of the convention.

Heated discussions followed the presentations of each LSD paper as the pro and anti-LSD elements vied to be heard. Several discussants from the floor eventually had to be asked to relinquish the microphone and return to their seats. Some called for the total abolition of all LSD use, including whatever research is still in progress. And LSD became an issue at some of the convention sections where it was not even on the agenda (e.g., the "Alcoholism" and "Suicide" sections).

On the other hand, some investigators defended LSD's use in research and therapy and claimed to have seen few adverse effects. One psychiatrist from another country claimed to have given patients up to thirty LSD treatments without any side effects. (When one of the contributors to this volume later questioned him, he admitted that some of his patients did become *psychotic* and others became *suicidal* and required hospitalization, but that these were not side effects but just part of "working through the LSD experiences." Even what we would call *convulsions,* with tonic/ clonic movements and loss of consciousness were regarded as part of the "abreactive experience" and not side effects of the drug.) One wonders if this investigator would call death by suicide an adverse effect.

Finally at the 7:30 A.M. Breakfast Panel on LSD on the final day of the convention (which I moderated) every seat was filled. The panel format immediately had to be discarded because the panelists refused to even consider their *scheduled* topics. Rather, two of the contributors to this volume confined their remarks to eloquent (if understandably defensive) pleas for the continuation and resumption of research such as they had been doing and for a decrease in the hysteria about LSD.

Such is the atmosphere of LSD work in this country at this time. One of our contributors has recently even lost his public health job, in large part because of his views on drug abuse and how to decrease it. I personally have had the one pharmaceutical company with the experience and equipment to analyze LSD refuse to analyze my samples out of (apparently unjustified) fear of reprisals from the Government. Representatives of another drug company which manufactures a tranquilizer used to combat LSD-induced side effects approached two of the contributors to arrange a panel on treatment of LSD-induced side effects. They soon withdrew their offer, again because of possible difficulty from Federal agencies. The representatives told us that they were receiving many requests from physicians all over the country about tranquilizer usage and dosage schedules to use in combating the LSD side effects. They added that these requests would now have to be answered with a "no comment" type statement.

Many physicians who work in medical and psychiatric emergency rooms have been horrified at the way some LSD researchers so glibly dismiss the drug-induced problems which pour in.

They easily explain the problem thus: "he had a conflict with his mother," "obviously pre-schizophrenic," "borderline," "not our fault," "nothing to do with the LSD."

Well known are the institutes for psychedelic research which have sprung up where (among other things) raters are used who take LSD themselves. Well known also is the now classic "experiment" where psilocybin was given to prisoners and the recidivism rate was studied with encouraging results—until the experimental design revealed that the drug group received many other benefits *besides* the drug which the control group did not.

If this is the way professionals and adults alike are responding to the drug problem (and the hippy drug users are just as nonsensical in their advocacy and support of the "drug scene") the prospects for LSD are dismal indeed. The generation gaps gets greater and few bridges are being built between the generations.

In summary (my views) LSD *can* teach us much. Research *must* resume—*good* research conducted by objective researchers, not by researcher/LSD users and not by LSD researchers whose entire careers depend upon proving the beneficial effects of the drug. Hysteria must diminish. We in the professional community have an especially important role. When we abandon objectivity and attribute all adolescent drug use to a Communist plot, to pornography, to an "eloquent Vietnam protest" or whatever our favorite hobbyhorse, we do our youngsters a great disservice. Likewise, when we overly identify with the adolescents, rail against the "over thirty" generation, and mouth the anti-establishment "it's all the liquor lobby" mythologies, it only worsens the problem.

We must try to be objective and yet firm about what we have seen and believe about drugs. We must not change our views depending on the climate of our audience.

Opinion of Sidney Cohen

We are seeing a number of trends emerging, now that the psychedelics have been in lay use for half a dozen years. They may represent significant indications about the future of these agents, but at the moment only speculations are justifiable. The following currents and countercurrents are discernible at this time.

1. A number of people are taking LSD at infrequent intervals and continuing to pursue careers, accept responsibilities and support themselves and their dependents. Whatever use they are making of their occasional indulgence is not reflected in overt patterns of markedly altered behavior.

2. A fair number of people, many young, have "dropped out," forming foci of a hip way of life in the larger cities. The hip subculture is almost entirely a drug-taking one. The drugs are usually marihuana, LSD or DMT, but a vast assortment of other botanicals and chemicals are occasionally used. Of these, methedrine is the most popular. Three "heads" are known to me who have switched from LSD to methedrine.

3. A small group of acidheads have stopped using LSD. Some of them were LSD evangelists in the past; now they believe that the LSD way is not for them. Others have had bum trips or adverse reactions and these have dissuaded them from further usage.

4. Perhaps the largest group numerically consists of people who have used LSD once or a few times and whose reasons for taking the drug have been satisfied. They are not involved in LSD taking.

5. Some adolescents or young adults continue to be introduced to LSD usage. Most of them seem to turn onto this potent drug for trivial or frivolous reasons: for a high, to avoid frustrating life situations, to be part of an in group, or simply for a new kind of euphoric experience.

6. Human research with LSD has dropped off considerably. In view of the reports now appearing on the effects on cytogenetic structure, a further reduction is possible. At the time this is written, chromosomal alterations have not been demonstrated, in my opinion, in amounts ordinarily used with research subjects.

7. The legislation regarding LSD does not seem to have made an appreciable impact on the quantity available or the number of users.

From the tendencies noted above, it seems likely that the drug will continue to be taken by an unknown number of people. Eventually that number will decrease as it becomes less of a novelty and as many weary of the "being" way of life and drift back into the "becoming" way, just as most beatniks of the early 1950's became more or less reintegrated into the culture from which they had previously disaffiliated themselves.

Opinion of Joel Fort

The immediate future, perhaps the long-term future, appears bleak. The issues will remain polarized, extremism will breed extremism, and irrationality will continue to predominate. Police agencies will continue to expand their spheres of influence, budgets and personnel and will foster more drug use. The abuse of both legal and illegal drugs will continue to increase with considerable harm to the individual and to society. More potent LSD-type drugs will be synthesized and used indiscriminately. The unjust and inconsistent laws and the selective and harmful enforcement of these laws will continue and will bring about even greater problems for the individual and society.

The sensationalistic use of drugs as a technique for selling newspapers, building bureaucratic power, or winning elections will continue. Effective rehabilitation programs will be few in number and opposed by the rigid and narrow attitudes of the enforcement agencies. Those dangerous drugs (alcohol and tobacco) presently advertised and widely distributed will continue to be uncontrolled due to the political and financial power of the manufacturers of these drugs and the large tax revenues gained by their distribution. Human research projects will be few in number, generally very conventional or concerned with the applications of such drugs as LSD to chemical warfare, and impeded by an increasingly complex bureaucratic regulatory process.

In the M.A.D. world, drug use will continue to be used

as a smokescreen, scapegoat and anti-intellectual device by the establishment or power structure of the society, which will continue to enlarge the generation and creditability gaps by seeking oversimplified pseudosolutions and hypocritically avoiding the complex roots of this problem.

None of this should be surprising in a world perhaps on the eve of destruction (which is in large part the reason why so many people are "turning on" with either the old or the new drugs).

Opinion of Keith S. Ditman

LSD, being an extremely potent chemical changer of consciousness, is of utmost interest and importance. How does a molecule act in the brain in such minute amounts to alter awareness so profoundly? The answer to this question will be sought until it is found. It could tell us much about brain functioning and awareness. The potency and mechanism of action of LSD are intriguing considerations, but not the only ones for the future of LSD and other hallucinogens. The very nature of the psychological effect of LSD, and this is shared by the other hallucinogens, makes it a drug of great promise and problems. These drugs alter and increase the sense of awareness, so they are valuable tools in studying creativity, aesthetic appreciation and intellectual understanding. Not only do they intensify awareness, they also appear to alter or remove the mental defense mechanisms so that unconscious or unnoticed material can become conscious. These effects offer considerable hope in understanding, classifying and treating psychiatric conditions. For example, it is possible that psychotherapy can be made more effective and not so prolonged, that patients who need treatment, such as alcoholics, can be motivated to want it, and that more of the helpful and rewarding endeavors of man, such as philosophy, art, music and religion can be appreciated and utilized further, not just by the mentally disturbed, but by the normal and gifted as well. It is true that none of the reported uses of any of the hallucinogens—psychiatric treatment, aesthetic appreciation, psychological understanding, enhancement of certain intellectual endeavors and creativity, and parapsychological studies—have been conclusively established to be of value. But there are many encouraging reports indicating that this is possible. It has taken a long time and a lot of effort to understand and develop uses for radioactive materials. Understanding the effect and use of powerful drugs on the brain is no less simple a task. Unfortunately, progress is not made without a price, but one can learn from mistakes.

LSD has recently become widely known as a public health problem. It is being abused in nonmedical settings and by uninformed people. Unfortunately, this apparently will increase and continue. Ultimately, man will learn to control these substances and use them intelligently. This does not appear likely in the foreseeable future, however. LSD may not prove to be the drug for these new uses—it may be too toxic—but other drugs will be developed for the above uses.

Opinion of Duke D. Fisher

Recently a housewife informed me that LSD was the greatest threat to our national security since the Axis powers during World War II. A day later, a college student communicated his feeling that LSD is our last chance for world peace. It is unfortunate that few people are willing to attempt an objective appraisal of LSD without either seeing the drug as a malevolent agent or finding it to be a magical solution for any individual or social ill. Most drugs have some beneficial properties as well as undesirable side effects. It is on the basis of a careful assessment of both the good and harmful effects of the drug that it finds a place in medical usage. The same physician who readily prescribes an antihistamine or aspirin is more reluctant to prescribe a steroid preparation or powerful antibiotic unless there is a definite indication. When a patient is extremely sick with a malignancy, the physician is willing to use powerful chemotherapeutic agents possessing potent side effects. In other words, the severity of some illnesses demand the use of drugs for therapeutic benefit that may have accompanying deleterious side effects. The side effects from LSD are becoming increasingly apparent as the illicit use of the drug continues. Any therapeutic value that LSD may have must be weighed against the known serious side effects that have been mentioned in this publication. Intractable alcoholics and drug addicts are people for whom the need for some therapeutic tool may justify the risks of LSD. However, there is no conclusive evidence that LSD is in any way beneficial. If research can be encouraged and expanded, some of the beneficial aspects of LSD may be realized. If there are no therapeutic benefits from LSD, then it is important to be cognizant of this fact. Unfortunately, the proselytizers and cultists of LSD who curse legislation restricting its usage have done more to deter scientific research of LSD than any other group. Many legitimate researchers are reluctant to work with a drug that has been the focus of much hysteria and mystical claims. Some researchers, on the other hand, use LSD themselves and have difficulty being objective concerning the actual effects of the drug. LSD will not save humanity, nor will it destroy humanity. LSD is not magic; it is a powerful mind-altering drug which may have some limited psychiatric use. The persistent widespread usage of LSD in the name of mysticism, in the name of "kicks," or in the name of curiosity is not only dangerous to the LSD user but also perils legitimate research.

POSTSCRIPT

Why do youngsters take LSD? Many reasons have been given why youngsters in this generation are so oriented to marijuana, LSD, "uppers" (amphetamines), "downers" (barbiturates) and the like. These reasons range from peer-group pressure to be one of the gang, to curiosity and the desire to experience different things. Kicks or thrill-seeking are often implicated as a reason, as is the reaction against the disillusionment about the many imperfections in the adult world (living in the "world of the bomb"). Alienation has also been cited. Certainly the common feature and a core reaction, in my experience with drug users, is that of *rebellion*. When listening to the fantasies of the youngster as he smokes marijuana, one frequently hears that he is wondering "what Mom or 'teach' would think if they only knew." Some youngsters have even told me that they enjoy alcohol better, but that if their parents knew they were drinking they would be not at all dismayed and just think it was a joke. Thus, these youngsters do not use alcohol to rebel.

The struggles of adolescence, of course, provide us with clues as to the reason for taking drugs like LSD. First of all, particularly when using LSD, youngsters feel that they do not have any hang-ups with anger or sexual feelings. Adolescence is the time when youngsters have to work out these feelings (by sexual experimentation and angry rebellion at the adult world) in order to make an eventual adjustment as an adult. They must decide where they are going, who they want to emulate, and what they want to do in life.

At a lecture in Fresno a youngster stood up in the crowd and shouted that he would prefer to remain in his room drugged on LSD for the rest of his life than *ever* have one angry thought towards anyone. And, as one youngster put it so typically, "Why waste something as good as LSD on something as common as sex." Likewise, the attraction of the Haight-Ashbury section of San Francisco is, according to the multiple youngsters I have treated who have spent time living there, the way there are no obligations. People drift in and drift out, passing around bread and flowers but with no responsibilities for any one else. These relationships are casual and never mobilize the feelings of frustration, depression, etc. that one-to-one relationships occasion. However, the instinctual derivatives of anger and sexuality do manifest themselves despite the drug use. For example, we have seen angry destruction of city flower beds under the guise of peace and love in flower giving. Even the dependency conflict emerges, for many of the hippies apply for welfare and demand to be supported by the very adults whose way of life they repudiate.

There was a marvelous letter by a student in the UCLA *Bruin* last April 10, entitled "Love in not Love." In the letter the student so wisely wrote: "But to love is not to proclaim love, nor to illustrate it, nor to waffle about it, nor to make taken exchanges at the level of a three-year-old mentality. . . . Love, rather, is best expressed by acts of genuine kindness in the context of daily living and by one's unshakable sense of responsibility not only to the 'world,' not only to 'humanity,' but also to those who look to one for comfort and support and companionship, and to those who, by virtue of their having given these things already, stand deservedly in need of repayment. It is easy to emit 'love feelings' toward an inhibited young lady meditating on a log in the middle of a love-in."

Another characteristic of adolescence is the coexistence of extreme gullibility (the youngsters buy the nonsensical huckstering of a Timothy Leary) and sensitive perceptivity. Thus, they see through and react to the fundamental hypocrisies (that we adults perpetrate) with great disillusionment. For example, we try to tell them that it is okay for Mom to have her (amphetamine) diet pills and for Dad to take his tranquilizer every day so that he can stand his boss, and for all of us to have our cocktails each evening but that it is the *youngster's drugs* (their marijuana and LSD) that are bad. They reject this form of hypocritical reasoning.

What can we do? A new generation seems to have arisen— variously called beatniks, hippies and flower people. We adults seem to be at a total loss to cope with them. I recently heard of an encounter that beautifully illustrated the generation gap. It occurred between a San Francisco mounted policeman and a female hippie. The girl tried to give the officer a flower. He refused it. Then she tried to place the flower in the bridle of his horse. He became agitated and finally told her where she "could stick the flower." Her response—"Flowers are for giving, not sticking." What we can do to ease the generation gap, reflected so often by drug taking, is both a very difficult problem and also potentially a very solvable one. For it is now obvious that the law can't handle it, that today's family unit is exerting much less pressure on youngsters, certainly religion hasn't met the challenge, and psychiatry has not been very helpful either. Although these youngsters aren't really happy, they are rarely committed to working out their problems in a non-drugged way. The myth has spread that UCLA's Neuropsychiatric Institute somehow has magic answers to the problems of youth and drugs. People call from all over the country to try to hospitalize patients at our facility, but in reality we do very poorly with this age group. Even those youngsters who have come in with severe drug reactions often go out and return to drugs. Thus the task falls to (perhaps unwilling) educators, but even they are at a loss as to what to do. So much of the situation is that of youngsters *testing* adults and asking for *intelligent* limits and controls.

When we speak to youngsters about LSD, one sentence at the beginning of the presentation seems to make all the difference in the world. It is, "We have not been sent by your parents, the school administration, the police or narcotic officers, the American Medical Association, or the alcohol or tobacco interests to get you *not* to take LSD; we are merely here to present the facts so that you can decide for yourself." Then there is a lot of receptivity to what we say instead of rebellion. But the youngsters never really accept what we say until they have tested us during the question and answer period following the lecture. Typical questions that they usually ask include the following: 1) *How can you know anything about LSD or study it if you haven't taken it yourselves?* Our answer—We know lots of good obstetricians who have never had babies themselves. 2) *What about marijuana?* Our answer—This is a complicated question, but essentially we can say that no research has been done in this country in the past thirty years on the dangers of "pot." For whatever apparently inexplicable reasons, a marijuana offense is now a felony and you should be aware that an arrest can adversely affect your entire lives. 3) *What about smoking, alcohol and traffic accidents?* Our answer—These are really very, very severe problems in our culture, but for some reason we adults haven't chosen to consider them as problems.

It has been very interesting in our work with educators at all levels to note the wide variety in approach to the drug problem from school to school. We have lectured in some schools where there are very minor problems with drugs, and yet the administration wants to present the facts to the children and to open the topic up for discussion. On the other hand, for example, administrators at three high schools in well-to-do neighborhoods near our university have adopted the "ostrich policy." They pretend that no drug problem exists, although the narcotics officers periodically raid students, parents call us, and even the children write us letters beseeching us to lecture at their schools. Of course we are not invited in, no open discussion occurs, and drugs remain exciting and forbidden.

So many adults, when asked by their children about drugs, pound the desk and say, "It's bad because it's illegal and that is all you have to know." They don't read and they don't give the children any credit for perceptivity. Secondly, and this is unfortunately so often true particularly of narcotic officers, marijuana and LSD are often included together in one breath. However, they are as different as day and night. LSD is hundreds to thousands of times more deadly than marijuana. Thus, when the children are told that marijuana kills, they not only ignore that but they *also ignore everything* the adult says about LSD, figuring that they have been lied to anyway.

We adults often get defensive and try to defend society's other problems, like alcohol, traffic accidents and tobacco's harmfulness. We sometimes even try to suppress the proponents of LSD by censoring them and by making statements like "if you don't like the University the way it is, get out." However, much progress in society has come from rebellion and dissatisfaction. The tragedy in this case is that it is a *drugged rebellion.*

Adults must be informed about drugs, and we must talk to our adolescents about them; we must *not* resort to an ostrich policy. Teen-agers have to be allowed to search and even to rebel. But we have to retain control of the home, the classroom and the campus. Youngsters are also *asking* for controls and get frightened when the adult abdicates his role and responds with excessive permissiveness; for example, the Berkeley riots.

Even though the adolescent is not totally an adult, he has to be treated like one in many ways. We have to admit it if we believe that we adults have not done such a good job in society. All one has to do is look at our fantastic abortion and marijuana laws, our sexual attitudes, the entire topic of censorship, etc. to realize that we have not done so well and that the adolescent sees this. He won't buy the fact that long hair on boys is inherently evil or that "all the trouble with the younger generation" (as some of our California groups contend) is either due to the violence shown on television programs or to topless waitresses. Remember, children need to identify with an adult and they want to do this desperately. But they are also trying to find their own way and to become independent. Also, remember that with their perception mixed in with their gullibility, they won't blindly accept our authoritarian pronouncements anymore.

J. Thomas Ungerleider

INDEX